Men's Health®

PEAK CONDITIONING
GUIDES

ESSENTIAL
CHEST
&SHOULDERS

AN INTENSE 6-WEEK PROGRAM

BY

Kurt Brungardt

RODALE®

© 2002 by Kurt Brungardt

Illustrations © by Karen Kuchar
Photographs © by Rodale Inc.

Printed in the United States of America
Rodale Inc. makes every effort to use acid-free (∞), recycled paper (♺)

Interior and Cover Designer: Susan P. Eugster
Interior and Cover Photographer: Mitch Mandel/Rodale Images
Interior Model: Lance LaMar

Library of Congress Cataloging-in-Publication Data

Brungard, Kurt, 1964–
    Essential chest & shoulders : an intense 6-week program / by Kurt Brungardt.
        p.   cm. — (Men's health peak conditioning guides)
    Includes index.
    ISBN 1–57954–309–X paperback
    1. Bodybuilding.   2. Chest weights.   3. Shoulder exercises.   I. Title: Essential chest and shoulders.
    II. Title.   III. Series.
    GV546.5 .B78   2002
    613.7'13—dc21   2001004608

Distributed to the book trade by St. Martin's Press

2 4 6 8 10 9 7 5 3 1 paperback

Visit us on the Web at www.menshealthbooks.com, or call us toll-free at (800) 848-4735.

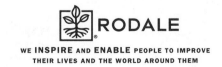

RODALE
WE **INSPIRE** AND **ENABLE** PEOPLE TO IMPROVE
THEIR LIVES AND THE WORLD AROUND THEM

CONTENTS

INTRODUCTION

I'm willing to bet you opened this book with a whole lot of optimism about building your chest, shoulders, and upper back. I'd even hazard a guess that you're shamelessly thrilled by the thought that you're just weeks away from a noticeably buffer upper torso.

As well you should be. I can't think of a more exciting project than the transformation of your own body into something bigger and better. Best of all, there's nothing risky or unhealthy about this particular adventure. Quite the opposite, in fact.

But it's an adventure that wasn't always so easily embarked upon. Sure, guys have been muscling up since *Homo sapiens* first pushed a boulder in front of his cave to keep out furry, razor-fanged predators. But until relatively recently, serious fitness training was perceived as an activity for, shall we say, borderline fanatics. The perception was cut-and-dried: Ironheads worked out. Regular guys didn't.

Even when the benefits of physical activity finally became too obvious to ignore, most of the attention focused on endurance workouts like running and cycling. Yes, more guys started getting into strength training, but more often than not, lifting weights was still misconstrued as a self-indulgent obsession for macho narcissists.

Not any more.

Muscle is mainstream now, for at least two very good reasons. One is the recent tidal wave of scientific proof that more muscle equals more health—not just for the chosen few but for everybody. Granted, a little harmless vanity may have something to do with your goal of a V-shaped upper body. But so might a lowered risk of disease, improved cardiovascular health, sounder sleep, increased energy, a richer sex life, and stabilized body weight—not to mention better-fitting clothes. All of that—and more—awaits you.

The other important development in the past decade or two is the advancement of exercise science. We know a lot more than we used to about how muscles get bigger and stronger. And all the new knowledge has actually led to less complicated workouts. Case in point: The Core Program you'll follow in this book is state-of-the-art, yet simple.

Author Kurt Brungardt knows all about groundbreaking programs. He's been at the vanguard of strength training for a couple of decades now. His breakthrough approach to midsection development earned him national renown as the consummate Man of Abs. You'll soon see that his expertise applies to building the rest of the body as well.

More important for you, Kurt has a special knack for communicating his know-how. So you'll have no trouble applying his expertise to your own body. If you're a veteran of the other two books in his *Men's Health* Peak Conditioning Guides series—*Essential Abs* and *Essential Arms*—you already know what I'm talking about. If you're starting out with this book, you'll soon see what I mean.

If I had to choose one adjective for Kurt's approach to upper-torso training, it would have to be *no-nonsense*. In the pages ahead, he delivers a straightforward, step-by-step presentation of what to do, how to do it, and why. No sugarcoating. No shortcuts. Just a clear explanation of a program that works.

Yes, the Core Program in this book is simple. Just don't mistake *simple* for *easy*. There's nothing quick and dirty about it. You have to "do" this book, not just read it. Kurt provides the theory, the program, and a lot of sound advice. You have to put in the effort.

Kurt and I are dedicated to the proposition that every guy deserves a rock-hard chest, speed-bump shoulders, and a world-beater upper back. And unlike in the old days, you don't have to wonder whether getting it is the right thing for you. It is. It doesn't matter whether you know your way around a weight room or have never before picked up a dumbbell. Whatever your level, if you want a bigger and stronger upper torso, *Essential Chest & Shoulders* will show you how to get it.

—*Lou Schuler*
FITNESS DIRECTOR
MEN'S HEALTH MAGAZINE

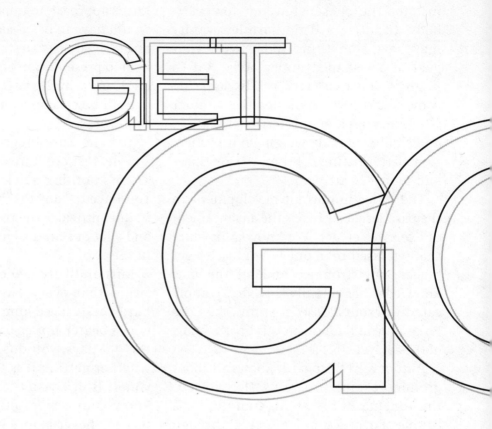

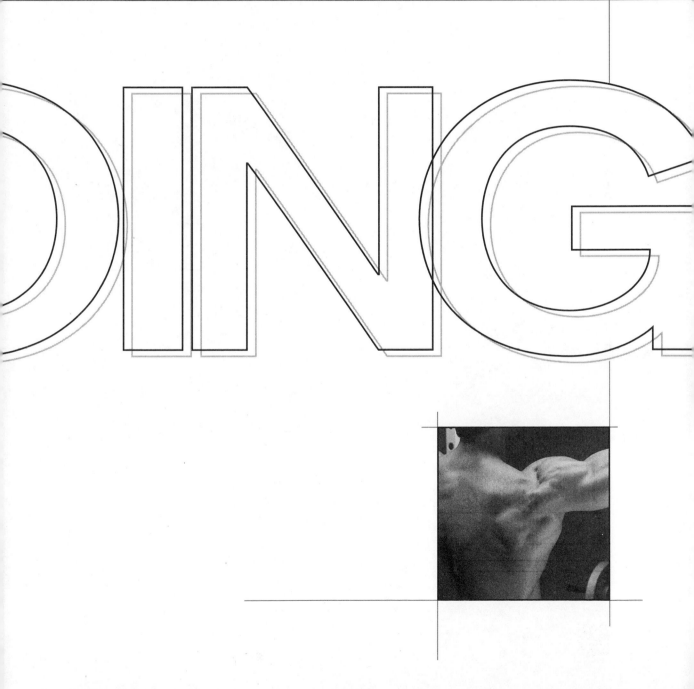

PART ONE

CHAPTER ONE

ESSENTIAL PLAN

Ever ask yourself why you want a bold chest, broad shoulders, and strong upper back? Oh, sure, there's health, strength, and a knockout appearance that'll get you places. Those things you'll reap in spades as you progress through the book.

But there's another, more anthropological reason: The chest is a body-language tool as old as the human species. The male chest-thrust has signaled dominance since Fred used it to remind Barney who the show was named for. And the high-tech modern man still communicates his pride with his chest (as does the high-tech modern woman, for different reasons).

The beauty of your soon-to-be-well-developed upper torso is that you won't have to go around thrusting out your chest to assert yourself. Your 24-hour pecs of steel will suffice to remind the world—and yourself—that you're a force to be reckoned with.

Essential Chest & Shoulders gets you there by taking you through a solid, well-rounded program that emphasizes upper-torso size and strength as it develops your entire body. The centerpiece is the 6-week Core Program that gets you pumping with the most productive exercises for your chest, back, and shoulders. You'll learn exactly how to do the lifts, how many to do, and when to do them.

At the same time, you'll be guided through the right kind of aerobic exercise, flexibility stretches, and dietary adjustments to complement your weight work. Once you've completed the Core Program, you'll feel new strength and see new muscle mass. Just as important, you'll have established a foundation for moving on to the more advanced exercises and routines in the final section of this book and for pursuing a plan for lifelong size and strength.

WHY THIS BOOK IS FOR YOU

If the Oakland Raiders' corps of linebackers call you up once a week for bodybuilding tips, this book probably is *not* for you. But if any one of the following describes you, keep reading.

The raw beginner. You never even thought about exercising until you looked up the word *concave* in the dictionary and saw that it described your sunken chest. Or maybe you realized too late that you weren't strong enough to carry your new bride across the threshold. The only thing you know about strength training is that you need to start from square one.

The procrastinator. You've been meaning to start working out but never quite got it together. You didn't know where to go or how to start. And besides, where would you find the time? And . . . hey, *Dirty Harry* is on TBS this weekend!

The lost soul. You've made the effort to get some muscle on your upper torso, but no go. You either followed programs that weren't right for you or you didn't have a program at all. You need some structure in your life, man.

The seeker. You love the results you've been getting from your diligent efforts in the gym. But now you're ready for something new. Or maybe you've followed the previous two books in the *Men's Health Peak Conditioning Guides* series—*Essential Abs* and *Essential Arms*—and decided it's time for your chest, upper back, and shoulders to catch up.

WHAT'S IN STORE

This book has four major sections. You're almost halfway through the first, which introduces the program and then explains what upper-torso training is all about, while dispelling some myths about chest, back, and shoulder development.

Part two lays down the groundwork for the actual program, running through the essential principles, techniques, and physiology underlying well-reasoned strength training. It also introduces the basics of the aerobic and flexibility routines you'll do.

Part three is the Core Program itself, presented in a step-by-step fashion that explains exactly how to do each exercise. The program is progressive, meaning you'll be asked to do a little bit more each week. (It's also presented progressively—you follow it by turning the pages one by one and doing what's outlined on each.)

Part four takes you beyond the Core Program, with maintenance strategies, more advanced exercises, and program-planning ideas that you can draw on for the rest of your life.

Along the way you'll be presented with:

- The basic upper-torso muscle anatomy
- The principles that will guide your strength training
- Essential techniques for doing the exercises correctly
- A stretching routine for better workouts and a more supple body
- A schedule for aerobic exercise that will improve your cardiovascular health without limiting your muscle gains
- A complete upper-torso strength-training program consisting of nine fully explained exercises
- Troubleshooting tips that address the most common problems and questions
- A total-body strength-training routine for overall development
- Nutritional advice to improve your workouts, reduce your body fat, and increase your muscle mass
- Advanced upper-torso routines

THE ESSENTIAL REQUIREMENT

There aren't any gimmicks in *Essential Chest & Shoulders*. No fancy gadgets. No secret sauce. The program is based on strength-training principles proven to build muscle mass in the upper torso, increase strength, and promote lifelong health. It's put together so that beginners who've never before touched a dumbbell can move through a steadily increasing workload and see gains.

As noted, the book provides step-by-step instructions accompanied by information to help you understand why you're doing what you're doing. Common questions also are answered along the way.

But you have to bring a little something to the party too: commitment. A good start is to start reading—all the way to the end. Skimming or picking out highlights won't cut it with a deliberately structured program like this one.

And, of course, you have to do the exercises. You have to keep doing them over the 6 weeks of the Core Program. If you're like most guys, you're going to love doing these routines. But make no mistake about it, there will be times, especially early on, when you'd just as soon skip those last three sets and get home in time for the opening face-off. Or maybe you'll be tempted to write off a day's workout altogether.

That's when commitment kicks in. That's when you have to remember that the difference between ordinary schmoes and studs who pop the buttons off their dress shirts just by taking a deep breath is in how they handle these times. The streets of Flab City are paved with the bones of guys who caught the opening face-off.

But you already know that. That's why you're reading this book. With your rock-solid commitment, you're on your way to a rock-solid upper torso.

So let's rock and roll.

CHAPTER TWO

ESSENTIAL
FACTS

Some folks connect the classic V-shaped male torso with caricatures of mythic heroes like Tarzan or Hercules. Or they associate it with the excesses of elite bodybuilders who earned their bold-faced Vs at the price of living regular lives. Either way, they don't consider it normal.

But the fact is that a shape resembling an inverted pyramid from the small of the back to the shoulder blades is the natural result of healthy mid- and upper-body muscle development. A male body with taut abs, a minimum of body fat, and strong muscles in the chest, back, and shoulders is going to have that shape.

That's why it's the classic ideal. That's why women like it. That's why we want it. And that's what this book aims to help you achieve.

WHAT MAKES IT LOOK LIKE THAT?

Take a look at the rear view of one of those human-skeleton charts that science teachers keep rolled up over the chalkboard. Just above the pelvis, the only bone you see is the spinal column, in the middle. But going up, the bone mass fans out with the rib cage, creating the lower part of a V.

Then, just when the rib cage starts circling back in, the outward diagonal trend is taken over by each scapula (shoulder blade) and culminates with your outer shoulders, where your clavicles (collarbones) sits over your the top ends of your humeri (upper-arm bones). The V is complete.

Now look at a muscle chart. As you'll see in chapter 4, the musculature of your upper torso is perfectly oriented to accentuate that V shape. Your biggest back muscle, the latissimus dorsi, runs diagonally in each direction from your hips, middle spine, and lower ribs to your armpits. In other words, this is a V-shaped muscle to begin with.

Now go outside and check out some guys (just this once). Where are all the V shapes? Chances are, they're hidden under the body fat that men tend to deposit in their bellies and chests, creating an apple shape. Or the Vs are disguised by small and flaccid muscles and weak posture; when shoulders slump forward, the triumphant V becomes a defeated question mark.

Any of those configurations—big gut, soft muscles, sagging posture—is unnatural. What's natural for a healthy man is broad shoulders tapering down to a narrow waist. That's what you'll work toward as you combine weight-training exercises with some aerobic work and diet adjustments. In a sense, the work you'll do won't create a V shape for your torso but rather will liberate and then accentuate the V shape that's already there.

MYTHS AND FACTS

The strange belief that a noticeably muscular, V-shaped torso is the exclusive domain of freaks and narcissists is just one

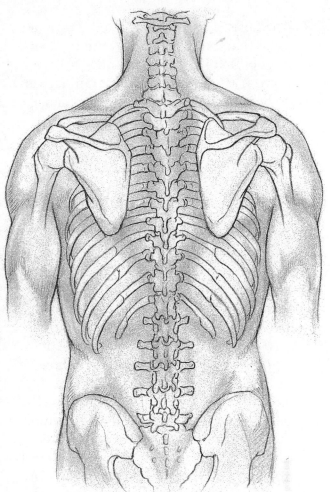

of many misconceptions that discourage some guys from going for it. So a good first step may be to debunk some of the myths about upper-torso development. Let's set the record straight now so you can move ahead.

Myth: It takes many long workouts with lots of exercises and dozens of sets to develop a big, multi-muscled area like the upper torso.

Fact: You'll do better with two weekly 45-minute upper-torso workouts, none with more than nine exercises or 18 sets.

The Core Program actually starts with less than that, building up to those numbers. It's not that I'm going easy on you. On the contrary, I designed the program for you to be able to work very hard on a manageable number of exercises.

True, your chest, upper back, and shoulders have lots of significant muscles that need to be worked. But the exercises you'll do hit several muscles at a time, often from more than one of these three body parts. More important, gains come from the kind of focused effort that can't be maintained over longer, more set-filled sessions. Intensity over volume—it's a guiding principle I'll repeat a lot in this book.

Myth: Doing more than one set of an upper-torso exercise is a waste of time.

Fact: The popular theory these days is that one set of any exercise will get you the same benefits as two or three sets. But it's still a leap to conclude that a second set is a waste of time. For one thing, the one-set theory is subject to debate, and among exercise physiologists, there are at least as many multi-set advocates as one-setters.

But even if the theory is correct, it presupposes a single set intense enough to fatigue the muscle as much as three sets would. Few guys—especially beginners or re-starters—are going to get that kind of intensity into a set, no matter how hard they try. So the Core Program starts off each exercise with one intense set and then adds a second set to make sure you exhaust the target muscles thoroughly.

Myth: Chest work doesn't burn midsection flab the way ab work does.

Fact: They both "burn" midsection flab equally—which is to say, not at all. Any reduction in body fat will take place wherever your body is programmed to shed it, regardless of where you focus your exercise. Despite the wishful thinking of millions of credulous crunchers, you can't target weight loss in a specific body part such as your belly by working the nearest muscle. If you could spot reduce like that, Rush Limbaugh would have skinny jaws from talking so much.

It's true, though, that men tend to store excess body fat in their bellies and chests, so beneficial fat loss is likely to show in those places. But that won't be because you did extra ab or pec work in your strength-training routines.

Besides, weight training is an anaerobic activity, so it doesn't "burn fat" (that is, use it for energy) the way aerobic exercise does. It does, however, result in a reduction of body fat over time, along with an increase of muscle mass. That in turn helps with weight management, since muscle speeds up your metabolic rate, or the number of calories you burn throughout the day and night.

It makes sense to take advantage of this program's weight training, aerobic exercise, and nutrition adjustments as a way of reducing body fat, rather than trying to lose weight, per se. A calorie-deficit diet at this time would hamper your efforts to grow your muscles.

Myth: All that muscle mass in the upper torso will make me muscle-bound, inflexible, and slow.

Fact: Current research has pretty much

put that old saw to rest. Weight training has no negative effect on flexibility. Even hard-core bodybuilders and weight lifters, whom many assume to be walking definitions of "muscle-bound," are really among the most flexible of athletes.

The Core Program will probably even increase your flexibility since you'll perform movements through a full range of motion for perhaps the first time in your life. And, of course, you'll do flexibility stretches, as outlined in chapter 5.

As for "slow," I've got two words: Carl Lewis. Here's somebody who was the fastest man in the world for about a decade, and his upper torso was just killer. All in all, sprinters make for pretty good role models as you pursue your upper-torso development. These are guys who spend a significant part of their training time lifting weights because they know muscle makes them faster.

Myth: Because of genetics, I can never make my chest strong and big.

Fact: Yes, some of us are born with fewer muscle fibers than others. Everybody has his own limit on upper-torso development. Your mission, should you decide to accept it, is to work toward reaching your own genetic potential. That's all anybody can ever do.

It doesn't make sense to not do something just because somebody else can do it more. Especially when the payoffs are so great. Anyone, no matter what his genetic destiny, can build enough new muscle to feel better, be stronger, live healthier, and look great.

Myth: Seeing results from an upper-torso program requires a lot of hard work and drudgery.

Fact: Hard work, yes. Drudgery, no. If you approach your upper-torso strength routine as a chore to be gotten through, odds are, you won't work intensely enough to make it worthwhile. You'll be like those pathetic people you see in every gym who slouch through their routines with no intensity and terrible form, trying to get through their workouts just because they think they're supposed to. If you take that attitude, you may as well return this book now for a full refund, because you probably won't stick with the program in the first place—and even if you do, you won't get the results you want.

Instead, you want to go about your workouts in a zone of high concentration, with a positive attitude and a controlled enthusiasm that borders on quiet joy. After all, you're improving your body, the only thing in the universe that's really yours. (Remember, unless you're a cosmetic surgeon, your own chest is the *only* one you can make strong and big.) What's not to like?

Fortunately, it's easy to get into that state of mind when you know you have a good program and you go into your first few workouts with energy and optimism. After that, when you realize you're starting to get stronger and feel better, you actually begin to look forward to your workouts and enjoy the hell out of doing them. That's when you start connecting with your body in more profound ways, and weight training becomes a permanent part of your life.

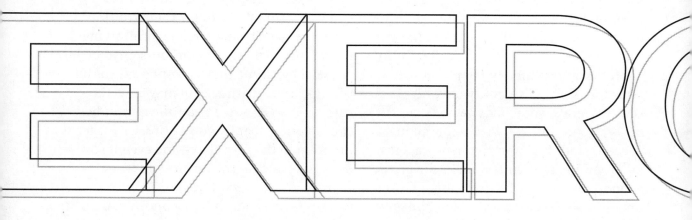

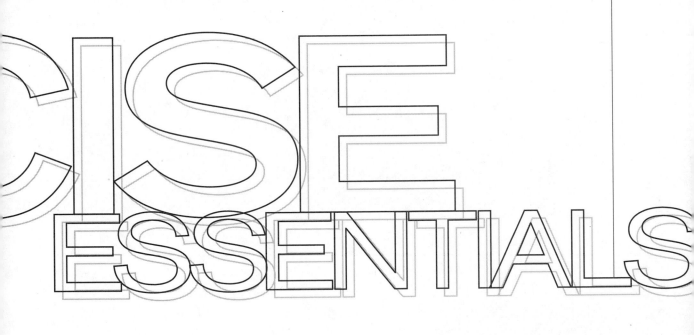

PART TWO

CISE
ESSENTIALS

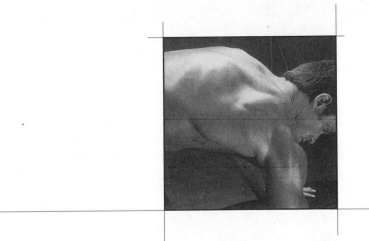

ESSENTIAL AEROBICS

Aerobic training is the best exercise for your numero uno chest muscle, your heart. At the same time, it's about as compatible with your goal of a big, bold upper torso as Hillary Clinton is with Jesse Helms on a blind date.

Catch a track meet on ESPN, and you'll get the picture. Sprinters (whose training is mostly not aerobic) boast V-shaped upper bodies that could land them on the cover of this book. Aerobically trained long-distance runners look like Pee-Wee Herman impersonators. Don't get me wrong, I admire marathoners for the high-achieving athletes they are. I just don't want my chest to look like theirs. Neither do you, or you wouldn't be reading this.

But you don't want to deep-six aerobic work either. While strength training helps with weight management by improving your metabolism, aerobic exercise is a far more efficient calorie burner. Most guys who achieve V-shaped torsos do it with a combination of weights and aerobic exercise. Just as important, aerobic exertion is the only sure-fire improver of overall cardiovascular health. Strength training doesn't guarantee that benefit.

You need aerobic workouts tailored to your needs as a man who's serious about a bigger chest, more imposing shoulders, and a stronger upper back. By following the aerobic guidelines given at each level of the Core Program, you'll claim the cardiovascular benefits without sabotaging your strength-training goals.

AIR SUPPLY

Short bursts of energy like lifting a weight are *anaerobic*, meaning "without oxygen." Your muscles do use oxygen but they don't get it from your lungs. Rather, it's freed up by chemical activity within the muscle itself. That internal supply doesn't last long before you have to stop and breathe hard to replenish it.

In *aerobic* ("with oxygen") exercise, your muscles use oxygen that you steadily breath into the lungs. Your heart then pushes that O_2 through your bloodstream to your muscles. Though you can't exercise at maximum intensity this way, you can work for long periods of time. That's why most popular endurance activities—cycling, running, swimming, cross-country skiing, aerobic dancing—offer excellent cardiovascular benefits.

THE IDEAL RATE OF RETURN

The long-term benefits of aerobic exercise come when you work at between 65 percent and 85 percent of your maximum heart rate. The easy way to estimate your maximum heart rate is to subtract your age from 220, the number that, theoretically, is the redline of a human heart, per minute. Say you're 40 years old. Subtract that from 220. Your maximum rate is 180. Sixty-five percent of 180 is 117. Eighty-five percent of 180 is 153. So you need to run or bike or swim at an intensity that makes your heart beat 117 to 153 times per minute.

This formula is accurate for probably about 60 percent of the population. Older guys could have higher beats per minute than the maximum predicted. Younger guys could have lower maximums.

Fortunately, you aren't training for the Olympics, so you don't have to be completely accurate. But that discrepancy is why many exercise scientists recommend that you monitor exertion rather than heart rate. Exertion during exercise can be measured by how hard you breathe and your ability to carry on a conversation. At the bottom end of the aerobic range, you can breathe steadily and keep up conversation. When you get to the top of the range, your breathing is still steady but is also deep, and talking is limited to one or two syllables. When your breathing is labored and you can't speak beyond a grunt, you've likely moved out of the aerobic-training zone and into anaerobic exercise.

THE LONG AND SHORT OF IT

The American College of Sports Medicine recommends a minimum of 30 minutes of aerobic exercise 3 days a week, with 20 of those 30 minutes spent in your aerobic-training zone. That's also the ideal maximum for anyone trying to build muscle, because serious cardio work and serious strength training cancel each other out. Your body doesn't know which to respond to when you pursue both.

Since the muscle-building stimulus is the one you want your body to heed, you'll devote the majority of your energy to strength training by doing the Core Program. You'll also do three 30-minute cardio workouts, either after you lift weights or (preferably) on separate days.

ESSENTIAL PHYSIOLOGY

Unlike your arms or abdomen, there's nothing simple about the musculature of your upper torso. Your chest, shoulders, and upper back are home to more than a dozen symmetrical pairs of major muscles that work together in intricate ways.

Fortunately, you don't need to pass an anatomy test to get all those muscles stronger and bigger. You just need to do the exercises in this book. But you'll do them much more effectively with a little bit of knowledge about which muscles you're actually working. Here's a primer on the most important ones in the upper torso.

YOUR MUSCLES

Pectorales major. These are the big guys, the chest broadeners, the pair you're usually referring to when you talk about building muscle mass in your chest. Each pec starts in the middle of your torso, where it's connected to (from top to bottom) your clavicle, sternum (breastbone), and upper ribs. From there, it spans your chest and inserts itself into the humerus, or upper-arm bone.

Each pec is a single muscle that's divided into upper and lower parts, or heads. To work both the upper (or clavicular) and the lower (or sternal) pecs, the Core Program exercises come at your pecs from different angles.

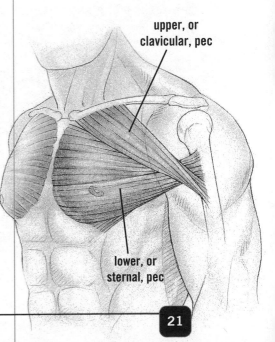

upper, or clavicular, pec

lower, or sternal, pec

Deltoids. They're your main shoulder muscles. The deltoids cap the shoulder girdle formed by the clavicles and the scapulae. Each delt attaches in three different places, creating three different heads. The exercises you'll do are designed to make sure you work all three heads: the anterior (front) deltoid, the medial (middle) deltoid, and the posterior (rear) deltoid. Well-developed delts give width to your shoulders and provide emphatic tips to the tops of your torso's V shape.

Rotator cuff muscles. Several smaller muscles rotate your shoulder in and out while helping to stabilize the joint. These are deep muscles that you rarely try to isolate during your workouts, although they assist in many of the exercises in the Core Program. The subscapularis is responsible for internal rotation of the upper arm and also helps with chest exercises, including the bench press. (It's located on the front of the torso, roughly opposite the infraspinatus.) The supraspinatus assists the

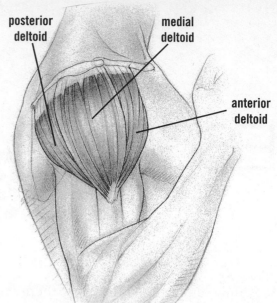

posterior deltoid

medial deltoid

anterior deltoid

deltoid in lifting your arm up and away from your body, and it's actually responsible for the first part of the motion in the lateral raise—the deltoids don't take over until the dumbbells are partway up. The infraspinatus and teres minor handle outward rotation of the upper arm. They have a minor role in exercises like the lat pulldown.

Trapezius. The two traps form a large flat diamond across your upper back, with points at the base of your skull, the back of each shoulder, and a spot about halfway down your spine. Named for the trapezoid shape, they're variously considered back, neck, or shoulder muscles. Along with a set of muscles called the rhomboids, the traps pull your shoulder blades together in back, which is a part of many exercises, including the rows you'll do in this program. (The deadlift, a powerlifting exercise, also involves pulling your shoulder blades together in back.) Another trap movement is lifting your shoulder blades up toward your ears, as in

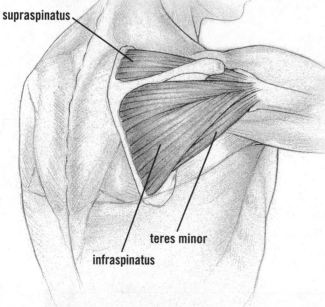

supraspinatus

teres minor

infraspinatus

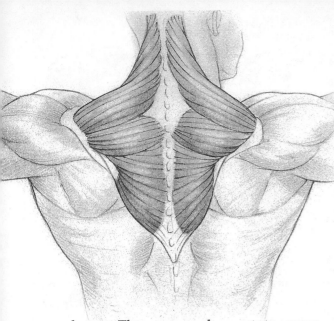

back, while the upper lats grow into "wings" that accentuate the V shape.

The latissimus dorsi is the largest upper-body muscle—so large that no single exercise works all of it. You'll hit it three ways in the Core Program.

BODY MECHANICS

You use your chest, upper-back, and shoulder muscles mostly for upper-arm movements that originate from your shoulder joint—motions such as throwing, pushing, waving, and blocking field-goal attempts. That presents a bit of a concentration challenge in your lifting, since most of us tend to pay more attention to our biceps or triceps whenever an exercise involves the arms, even if the target muscle is in our chests, backs, or shoulders.

You'll conquer that tendency as you gradually learn what it feels like for, say, your latissimus dorsi to lead the way (as in the lat pulldown) or for your pectorales major to work hard (as in the bench press). To help you get to that point, here's a rundown of the major upper-torso muscles' most important roles.

a shrug. The traps also rotate your shoulder blades upward (as in a shoulder press) and downward (as in a lat pulldown or pullup).

Latissimus dorsi. The pair of lats meet below the center of the spine, and each veers diagonally up your back toward your armpit so that together they form a V. Strong lower lats bring definition to your sides that's visible from front or

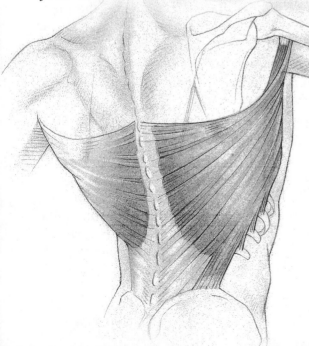

Pectoralis Major

What you do: Not many of us have ever actually thrown a discus, but those who have, used their chests to do it. That inward movement of the arm along a horizontal plane toward a point out in front of you (called *horizontal adduction*—a good thing to know if you ever find yourself in a kinesiology exam) is powered by your pectorals, with help from your front del-

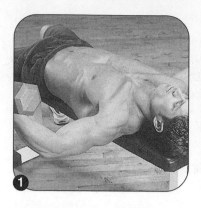 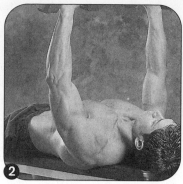 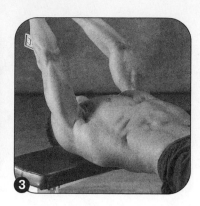

toids. The dumbbell fly (1) is the standard gym version of this movement. The bench press (2), the most popular chest-building exercise, combines two actions: horizontal adduction and shoulder flexion (pushing your arms out in front of you when they're down at your sides).

Other pectoral muscles: The *pectoralis minor* lies beneath the pec major. Instead of being connected to the humerus, it attaches to the shoulder blade and helps rotate it downward. Let's say you pick up a child off the floor and lift him over your head. Your shoulder blades rotate downward as your arms go up, an action made possible, in part, by your pecs minor.

The *serratus anterior* is another chest muscle that attaches to the shoulder blade. (If your muscles are really well-developed and your body is extremely lean, this muscle looks like fingers along the side of your rib cage, just below the outside of your pecs.) It helps rotate the shoulder blade upward. So let's say that, instead of lifting that child off the floor, you're pushing him on a swing. As you push down, your shoulder blades rotate

up, activating your serratus muscles. In the gym, the pullover exercise (3) duplicates this movement.

Deltoid

What you do: Ever see how Nazis saluted each other in those old war movies? Those guys were short on humanity, but they had shoulder flexion down. That's the movement of your arm straight up and forward to shoulder level. It's the work of your anterior (front) deltoid, with help from the upper pecs. (Above shoulder level, however, the trapezius takes over from the deltoid.)

Shoulder flexion is used in the front raise, an exercise you'll meet in an advanced program in chapter 13. But few guys really need extra work for their front delts. These muscles get plenty of work on chest exercises, particularly the bench press. They also work hard on the shoulder press. In fact, many veteran gym rats are overdeveloped in their front delts and underdeveloped in other parts of their shoulders since they spend more time on chest and shoulder work than on

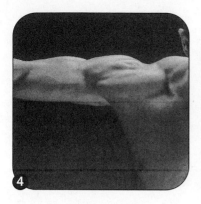
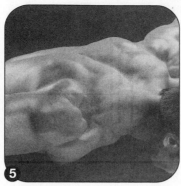
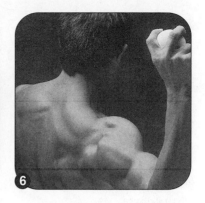

the muscles they can't see in the mirror. Rest assured, the Core Program will hit these muscles well enough.

Other deltoid actions: Don't forget, the three heads of your deltoids have different job descriptions. If the Nazis had saluted to the side instead of the front, they'd have used their middle deltoids to perform what's known as shoulder abduction. If they'd bent over to do the same thing, their posterior delts would've done most of the work. You'll do both in the form of lateral raises (4) and bent-over lateral raises (5), with no saluting involved.

Rotator-cuff muscles

What you do: Your rotator-cuff muscles spring into action during any arm movement that requires turning the humerus (upper arm bone) outward or inward. When you take your arm back to throw a baseball, you're using your infraspinatus, supraspinatus and teres minor muscles to perform external (outward) rotation. When you actually throw the ball (6), your subscapularis and teres major (a pair of small muscles in your upper back) per-

form internal (inward) rotation, with help from your latissimus dorsi.

Trapezius

What you do: When you shrug to indicate you don't know the answer to a question (or care about it very much), the upper part of your trapezius is lifting your shoulder blades in a motion known as scapular elevation. Assisting are some smaller pairs of back muscles—the aptly named levator scapulae, which roughly means "shoulder-blade lifters"—and the rhomboids.

Now, push your shoulders down (scapular depression) and it's your middle and lower traps doing the work, along with the pectoralis minor. This shoulder-lowering is included in a number of trapezius-taxing exercises, such as the lat pulldowns you'll be doing in the Core Program.

Another trap task is pulling your shoulder blades toward each other behind you, in an exaggerated military attention pose called scapular retraction.

Other trapezius actions: The trapezius has more to do with the position of your shoulders than arm movements, per se. But whenever you're working your arms above your head, you're using your traps. And your upper trapezius is also a neck muscle; it will tilt your head back for a view of skyscraper tops, and move it toward your shoulders.

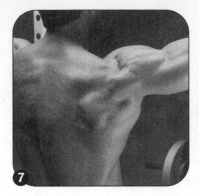 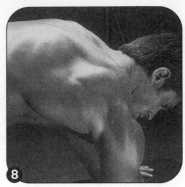

Latissimus Dorsi

What you do: Moving your raised arms downward toward the sides of your body is a job for your lats. If the motion is done with your arms starting in front of you, like a third-base coach commanding a runner to slide, it's called shoulder extension (the opposite of shoulder flexion). If it's done to your sides, parallel to your body, that's adduction (the opposite of the *ab*duction of the lateral raise, and not to be confused with the *horizontal* adduction of the fly or bench press).

A good example of adduction is the gymnast on the rings who starts with his arms extended to either side and parallel to the floor, and then elevates his body by pulling the rings straight down to his thighs. (There's one guy who doesn't need this book.) The lat exercises of the Core Program—pulldowns (7) and bent-over rows (8)—emphasize extension over adduction.

Other latissimus dorsi actions: Major League pitchers aren't always shining examples of the vaunted V-shaped torso, but they all have great lats. That's because the latissimus dorsi works with the subscapularis and teres major to perform internal rotation, a major component of throwing.

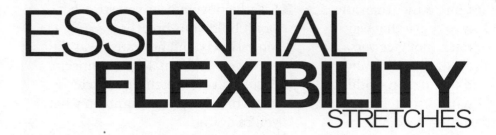

CHAPTER FIVE

ESSENTIAL FLEXIBILITY STRETCHES

My guess is that you're getting into the *Essential Chest & Shoulders* program because you want to be stronger and healthier, as well as look and feel better. Improving your flexibility helps with all those goals, and helps you get more out of your weight workouts. That's why the stretches presented in this chapter are a vital part of your Core Program.

The muscles you build while strength training won't prove particularly useful if they aren't flexible. Mind you, I'm not saying that weight lifting will make you less flexible; I've already said the opposite is more likely to occur— you'll get a little more flexible from lifting weights through a full range of motion. But doing targeted flexibility exercises will extend that range of motion, helping you train more efficiently and more comfortably. And you'll feel the benefits of increased flexibility 24 hours a day—at the gym, at work, at play, and in bed.

So blowing off flexibility work, as a lot of misinformed weight-trainers do, robs you of results. The stretching routine I'm prescribing for you is simple and should take less than 10 minutes. Believe me, it's worth it.

HOW TO STRETCH

The following 11 stretches hit all your major muscle groups, with special emphasis on the chest, shoulders

BENEFITS OF FLEXIBILITY

Increased range of motion

Improved sports performance and less risk of injury

More energy throughout the day from more efficient movements

Better posture, emphasizing the V-shape of your developing upper torso

Relief of muscle-joint stiffness, especially in older men

and back muscles that are the focus of your program. Follow these guidelines:

- Try to do your stretches just before your weight session, rather than after. You're less likely to skip it that way.
- Warm up to stretch, not vice versa.
- Stretch until you start to feel mild discomfort, and no further. Nothing is gained by forcing a stretch or pushing into pain; instead, you're creating an injury in your connec- tive tissues and compromising their integrity.
- Hold each stretch for 20 to 30 sec- onds.
- Breathe normally as you stretch. Don't hold your breath.
- Move slowly and hold steady at the extended position. Don't bounce.
- Focus on the stretching muscle as you work. Keep your mind on what you're doing.

Chest and Front-Shoulder Stretch

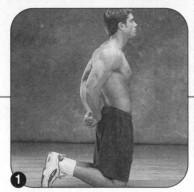
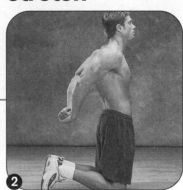

READY, SET, GO:

1. Kneeling, clasp your hands behind your back.
2. Slowly extend your hands up and back.

Upper-Trapezius Stretch

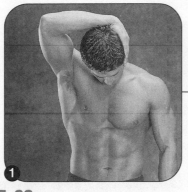 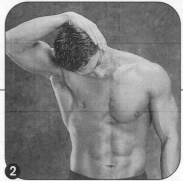

READY, SET, GO:

1. Drop your head forward, chin toward chest.

2. Place your right hand on the left side of your head, just above your ear. Lower your right ear toward your right shoulder, using your hand to gently assist. Repeat to the left, using your left hand on the right side of your head.

Horizontal-Flexion Series

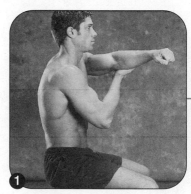 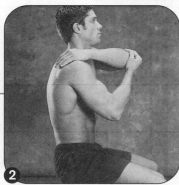 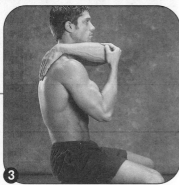

READY, SET, GO:

1. Extend your left arm across your chest past your right shoulder, using your right hand to extend the stretch. Be sure to keep the upper left arm chest-high. Don't bring the left shoulder forward or twist your torso. Switch arms and repeat.

2. Now reach behind your neck with your left arm, bending the elbow so your left hand goes behind your right shoulder. Grasp your left arm at the elbow with your right hand and use it to extend the stretch.

3. Walk the fingers of your left hand down your upper back as far as you can comfortably. Switch arms and repeat.

Deltoid Stretch

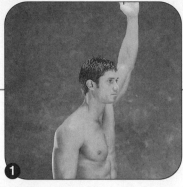 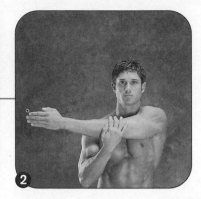

READY, SET, GO:

1. Extend your left arm straight up toward the ceiling, palm facing in.

2. Keep your arm straight as you lower it diagonally toward your right shoulder until it's parallel to your torso, shoulder-height. Use your right hand to increase the stretch, pulling gently at your left elbow. Switch arms and repeat.

External Rotation

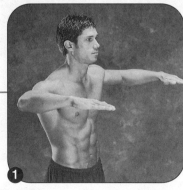 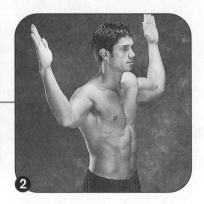

READY, SET, GO:

1. Hold your arms at shoulder level, your elbows bent so your upper arms are parallel to your shoulders and your forearms perpendicular to them, fingers pointed straight ahead.

2. Rotate your shoulder so your hands go back behind your shoulders without your upper arms or elbows moving. Continue the stretch as far back as comfortable.

Biceps and Forearm Flexor Stretch

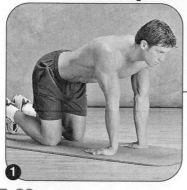 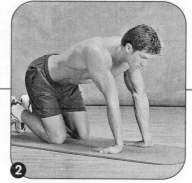

READY, SET, GO:

1. Kneel down with your arms on the floor in front of you and your fingers pointing back toward you.

2. Lean back until you feel a gentle stretch in your biceps and forearms.

Triceps Stretch

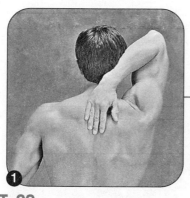 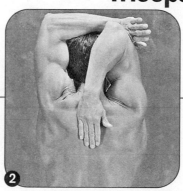

READY, SET, GO:

1. Lift your right arm so your elbow is bent next to your right ear and your right hand is toward the middle of your back.

2. Cross your left arm over your head so the back of your left hand lies against your right triceps muscle. Push back with your left hand until you feel a stretch in your right triceps. Switch sides and repeat.

Hamstring Stretch

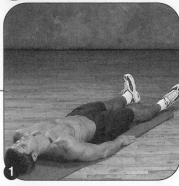 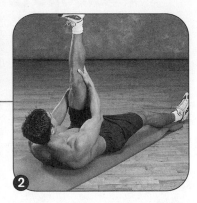

READY, SET, GO:

1. Lie on your back with your legs fully extended on the floor.

2. Lift your right leg and grab it with both hands, either above or below the knee, whichever is most comfortable. Gently pull it toward your head. You may find it helpful to raise your head and bring your chin to your chest. Switch legs and repeat.

Quadriceps Stretch

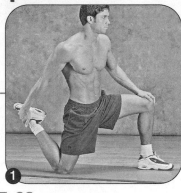 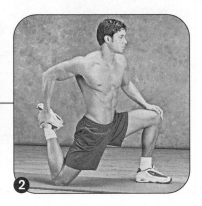

READY, SET, GO:

1. Kneel on your right knee with your left foot flat on the floor in front of you. Reach back and grab the top of your right foot.

2. Lean forward until you feel a gentle stretch in the front of your right thigh. Switch legs and repeat.

Lower-Back Stretch

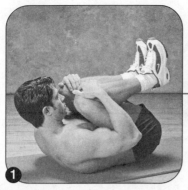 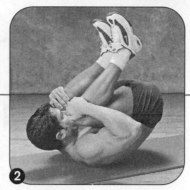

READY, SET, GO:

1. Lie flat on your back on a mat or well-padded floor and bring both knees up toward your chest. Grab both knees and gently pull them toward your shoulders as you tuck your head and bring your chin to your chest.

2. Now roll back and forth five times, gently and slowly.

Abdominal Stretch

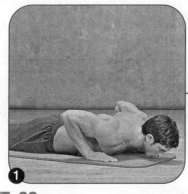 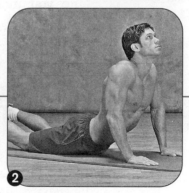

READY, SET, GO:

1. Lie on your stomach with your hands under your chest, palms down.

2. Slowly push up with your arms, arching your torso up. Keep your hips on the floor and look up.

6

ESSENTIAL PRINCIPLES

Getting the muscled chest, back, and shoulders you want isn't just a matter of following a series of instructions. Sure, we can show you how to flip some switches—lift this, stretch that—and it would work for a while. But if you want to truly benefit from strength training, you need to look behind the control panel and understand why the switches work the way they do.

Here are five basic principles behind strength training. Once you understand these, you'll understand how to get the best possible results, and enjoy the process of achieving them.

PRINCIPLE #1:
MUSCLES RESPOND TO STRESS

When your muscles are stressed by work that's harder than what they're accustomed to performing, they adapt by growing bigger and stronger. That way, the work won't be so hard the next time.

In the Core Program—or any good strength-training system—the work imposed on your muscles is progressively more difficult.

The most obvious way to increase difficulty is to steadily add weight. In fact, weight load and intensity are often synonymous in strength-training parlance. That's why you'll increase the weight you lift throughout the

Core Program. You'll also move up from one set of each exercise to two. And there'll be a new exercise for each muscle group every 2 weeks.

GROWTH COMES WITH RECOVERY

Your muscles don't grow while you're stressing them. It happens during the 24 to 48 hours after you leave the weight room, when your body adds protein to the muscle fibers to make sure they can handle the stress the next time around. This process is called hypertrophy. It will probably be a few weeks—and perhaps even 2 to 3 months—before you accumulate enough additional muscle protein to see a difference in your muscle size. But the process will occur if you give your body the right stimulus and enough time to recover in between workouts.

As a general rule, you want to give your muscles about 48 hours between workouts. So a Monday/Wednesday/Friday workout schedule works for most guys. In the Core Program, you'll work your chest, back, and shoulders 2 days a week—probably Monday and Friday—with a workout in between to hit your legs, arms, and midsection. This gives your upper-torso muscles 3 or 4 days to recover in between workouts, allowing you to lift with more intensity each time.

That sort of program is far beyond our mission here. If you're a beginner or intermediate lifter, you should see outstanding gains during the 6-week Core Program, and build on those gains using the advanced routines in chapter 13.

CONSISTENCY COUNTS

Stop training for any length of time and you'll lose your hard-earned new muscle mass a lot faster than you gained it. Many a frustrated strength-trainer has discovered the hard way that the muscle growth isn't permanent. Without extra stress, your muscles lose mass (a process called atrophy, the opposite of hypertrophy) because they no longer have any need to be big.

Consistency means commitment—a steady 2 or 3 days in the weight room, week in and week out. But commitment and fanaticism aren't the same thing. Your body and brain need downtime, and if you choose your breaks wisely, you'll make far better progress than if you never miss a workout. A good training program should include a week-long break every 4 to 12 weeks, with one or two longer breaks each year—2 weeks for Christmas and summer vacation, for example.

On the other hand, taking a month off for March Madness is a pretty bad idea, as is abandoning the gym from Thanksgiving to New Year's. A good exercise habit is self-perpetuating—you feel better, and want to maintain the good vibes. But inertia has some power, too. So plan your breaks, but also plan a quick return from those breaks.

PRINCIPLE #4:
EFFICIENCY PAYS

Efficiency, not longevity, is your guiding principle for productive workouts. With strength-training, more is not better. Better is better. If you're spending more than an hour in the gym on any given day, you're probably not working efficiently.

The efficiency principle calls for maximum focus and effort over a manageable number of sets and exercises. Emphasize good form to work the muscle properly. Use poundage that will fatigue your muscle at the end of one, two or three sets, rather than doing four or five or even more sets. Eliminate redundant exercises that work the same part of the same muscle. When you want to emphasize one set of muscles (as you've indicated by buying *Essential Chest & Shoulders*), split your workouts so you can focus all your energy on those muscles in one or two workouts a week, while still giving the other muscles the work they need.

The efficiency principle allows you to build the muscle you want without allowing your workouts to take over your life. The weight room is a nice place to be a few hours a week, but you don't want to have your mail forwarded there.

PRINCIPLE #5:
CONSISTENTLY CHANGE

There's a reason why the Core Program lasts 6 weeks instead of 6 months. A principle called periodization holds that your muscles respond best when presented with ever-changing challenges. You'll get plenty of that during the Core Program as the number of reps, sets, pounds, and exercises advances from week to week.

Eventually, though, even the best program will stagnate. Without more radical changes or a new program altogether, your muscle response will taper off, your motivation may deflate, and you can end up either overtraining or finding excuses to skip workouts. It's time to "periodize" your training and move beyond the Core Program. You'll learn ways to do that in part four of this book as you get into more advanced routines and a long-range plan for building an upper torso you'll be proud of.

ESSENTIAL
TECHNIQUES

There's enough tragedy in the world without more guys busting their buns in the gym only to see puny results. Unfortunately, it's a too-common story. Poor technique is often to blame.

Fact is, lifting weights doesn't come naturally. You have to make the effort to do it right. That said, it's not terribly difficult to learn proper technique. Here are the basics that apply to all weight-training exercises:

`#1`
ALWAYS WARM UP FIRST

For some inexplicable reason, the same guy who faithfully warms up before tennis, running, baseball, hoops—what have you—will burst into the gym and knock off a high-poundage set of bench presses before the door closes behind him. This guy's risking injury, because unprepared muscles and connective tissue strain and tear more easily. He's also limiting benefits; cold muscles simply don't work as efficiently as warm ones.

Warming up is a two-part process. The first part is literal: You want to increase your body's core temperature so the muscles can contract with greater force. Get this done with just about anything that moves your body—a few minutes on the treadmill or punching bag is enough. Cycling, jogging or briskly walking to the gym will also do the trick if you don't have too far to go. (A warmup should never turn into a workout. Tired muscles don't perform much better than cold ones.)

The second part is situational. You want to prepare your body for the specific exercises you're going to do. So before a bench-press set, you'd do a warmup set with a fraction of the weight you'd use to build muscle—maybe 50 or 60 percent. This forces blood into the muscles you're going to use, and also prepares your shoulder and elbow joints for the harder work ahead. (The joints secrete a lubricant called synovial fluid to help them work smoothly. It works like motor oil on your car's pistons.) Rest for a minute after this warmup set, then get to work.

GO SLOW

How fast you do the repetitions influences how fast you build muscle. For the Core Program, you want to stay on the slow side, especially as you lower the weight at the end of the lift. Count off in your mind a 1-second lift, a pause at the top, 2 or 3 seconds of lowering and a pause at the bottom before repeating.

Your goal is to maximize the amount of time your muscles are under tension, while still using a weight heavy enough to increase strength. If you do your repetitions quickly, your muscles don't spend much time under tension, and you end up using momentum and gravity to do much of the work.

In fact, when your goal is to build muscle, you should look at your workouts as "weight lowering" rather than weight lifting. That part of the lift—called the negative or eccentric contraction—induces the greatest damage to your muscles, and thus the greatest stimulus to build bigger ones. Remember, the reason your body makes muscles bigger is to avoid further damage. Your body always wants the next workout to be easier than the last one.

As you get more advanced you can alter your repetition speed to get different results. For example, when you move up to heavier weights, you have to do those repetitions faster—say, 4 or 5 3-second repetitions instead of 8 to 10 6-second reps. Your goal in that type of program isn't muscle mass so much as pure strength.

Some sports-training programs require sets of very fast repetitions with very light weights—perhaps three repetitions in 3 seconds with a weight that's just half your maximum in that lift. Those sets are designed to teach the muscles to move fast, not build bigger muscles.

At the opposite end is the Super Slow technique, in which you might do repetitions lasting 10 to 20 seconds. Whether or not Super Slow works is a subject of much debate. Most trainers believe the concept takes a good idea—lifting weights slowly—and moves it beyond the point of practicality and usefulness for most guys. When you lift and lower the weight slowly, you're teaching your muscles to contract slowly, which isn't what you really want them to do. And when you extend each repetition that long, you have to use weights that are too light to increase your strength. They probably won't do much for your muscle mass, either, despite the fact you're putting your muscles through extended time under tension.

For the Core Program, stick to the middle ground. You'll develop good form, build muscle fast, and increase your strength.

WORK IN YOUR FULL RANGE OF MOTION

Do every repetition until you reach maximum contraction and extension—as far up and as far down as it is comfortable and safe to go. That's the only way you're going to grow the entire muscle instead of just part of it. It also allows you to better put your muscle gains to work out in the real world—in sports, work, and recreation. And your range of motion might even increase as you continue to weight-train and do flexibility exercises.

Other than ignorance or laziness (which surely don't apply to you), the usual reason guys fudge on their range of motion is because they're using too much weight. Obviously, you can lift more if you lift it a shorter distance. But if you want a properly developed upper torso, stick to weights that allow a full range of motion. Doing half an exercise with twice the weight is still doing half the exercise.

STAY TENSE

A weight exercise challenges your muscles every inch of the way, and those inches don't all feel the same. The angle of movement changes, gravity comes into play in different ways, and the muscles themselves perform differently at different points of the lift. To take full advantage of every repetition, it is absolutely essential that you keep your target muscle tensed throughout the range of motion.

It's also important to pause at the top and bottom of the movement, when your muscle is fully contracted or fully stretched. At the top of the movement, a pause forces your muscles to work harder (they may even shake), creating a greater muscle-building stimulus. A pause at the bottom, when the muscle is fully stretched, forces your muscles to begin the next repetition with no "bounce." That is, you take all momentum out of the lift and force your muscles to push or pull the weight from a dead stop. Again, that makes the lift harder and thus more beneficial.

STABILIZE

When you play sports, you don't spend a lot of time trying to make muscles work in isolation. You want them to work together, making your movements fluid and efficient. But when you're trying to build muscle, you have to isolate your muscles. For example, if you're doing a standing shoulder press, you want your shoulders and arms to do the work, even though it would be easier to use your lower body to help generate momentum to get the weight moving. "Easier," though, means less beneficial to the muscles you're trying to build with the lift. Your goal is almost always to make the exercise harder, as long as it's still a safe and sane lift.

The key to keeping these other muscles out of the exercise is stabilization. Before starting an upper-body lift, you have to make sure your midsection and lower body are in a fixed, stable position. On a standing shoulder press, that means pulling in your abdominals to form a tight sheath around your middle, and bending your knees slightly to keep your body from swaying back and forth during the lift.

#6

FOCUS ON THE TARGET MUSCLE

Few upper-torso exercises isolate a single muscle group. A simple lat pulldown—an exercise so basic they even have old ladies doing it—uses muscles in your upper back, middle back, shoulders, upper arms, lower arms, and even in your chest. With all that going on, it's crucial to focus on the muscles you're *targeting* in the lift, rather than leaving it to your body to sort out.

You do that first by lifting the weight slowly, as discussed above, and imagining that the muscle you're targeting is doing the job by itself. Another trick is to imagine the muscles squeezing an object

at the end of the lift. For example, during a row or lat pulldown, imagine that your back muscles are crushing a can resting on your spine. On a chest exercise, pretend your pecs are squeezing a sponge that's sitting on your breastbone. These little visualization tricks help you concentrate on fully contracting the targeted muscle on each repetition.

Here's another trick to use on pulling exercises: Many people complain that they feel lat pulldowns and rows work their arms more than their backs. That's because they start the exercise by consciously pulling with their hands and arms. Instead, imagine that your hands are hooks, rather than animate, flexible body parts. When you pull the bar toward you on pulldowns and rows, imagine that your back muscles are pulling on hooks. In other words, consciously start the exercise with your back muscles, then finish it by using the can-crushing trick described above. You'll feel your back muscles in action from start to finish, and it won't be long before the results will be noticeable.

#7

BREATHE

Pay attention to your breathing until it becomes second nature as you lift. It should be rhythmic, usually at the rate of one full breath per repetition. The preferred procedure is to inhale before the first repetition, then exhale as you go up and inhale again on the way down.

But the main thing at first is to breathe,

Just as a pitcher's grip on the ball has a lot to do with how that pitch moves on its way to the strike zone, the way you grip the dumbbells will determine which muscle fibers get worked.

The three dumbbell grips are:

1. Underhand. **Your palms face forward (away from your body) in what's called a supinated grip.**

2. Overhand. **Your palms face backward in what's called a pronated grip.**

3. Neutral. **Your palms face each other.**

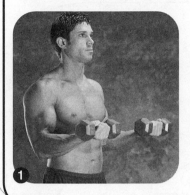
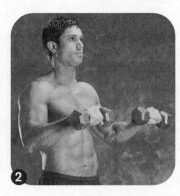
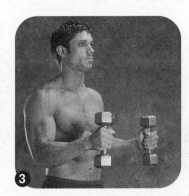

period. Beginners tend to hold their breath, sometimes for all the reps. Such a distraction leads to rushed sets, bad form, and an unwanted spike in blood pressure.

#8
FOCUS ON FORM

Every exercise in this book comes with specific instructions for doing it right. Points that may strike you as trivial at first—grip type, palm orientation, head position, foot placement, back alignment—determine how your muscles are going to work. If you ignore them, you're sacrificing benefits.

Obviously, no panel of judges is going to give you style points for doing it right. The good form allows you to get the best possible results in the least amount of time, and keeps from you losing time to pain and injury.

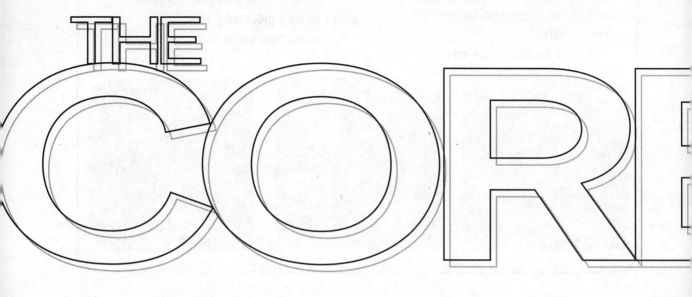

PART THREE

PROGRAM

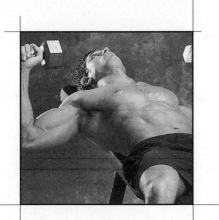

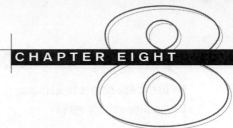

CHAPTER EIGHT

ESSENTIAL KNOWLEDGE

Throughout the 6-week Core Program, you'll lift weights three times a week. Two of the sessions target your chest, shoulders, and back. The third hits your lower body and midsection for overall body development.

In Level One, you'll do just three upper-torso exercises—one each for your chest, shoulders, and back. You'll continue to do these throughout the Core Program. At Level Two, you'll add another exercise for each of the three upper-torso parts, then a third at Level Three. Besides adding new exercises, you'll increase the total number of sets at each level and increase your weights as you go.

You'll do the same three lower-body exercises every week, working up to three sets of each. The two midsection exercises will change in each level since your abdominal muscles are smaller and adapt faster.

By week 6 of the Core Program, you'll do 18 sets in your upper-torso workouts. That's a 45-minute workout, max. You'll end up strength training about 2 hours a week. Add the three half-hour cardiovascular sessions and that's 3½ hours of exercise per week. That's enough to achieve maximum results without discomfort, frustration, or injury.

PERFORMANCE TIPS

To help you get the most of the exercises, you'll find performance tips accompanying each new exercise. While

Use these charts to help you monitor your progress through the Core Program. In the "Workout" columns, the numbers on the left sides of the slashes are the recom-

	WEEK 1	
LEVEL-ONE EXERCISES, MONDAY AND FRIDAY	**WORKOUT 1**	**WORKOUT 2**
Dumbbell bench press	1 set, 10–15 reps/	1 set, 10–15 reps/
Bent-over dumbbell row	1 set, 10–15 reps/	1 set, 10–15 reps/
Rotation press	1 set, 10–15 reps/	1 set, 10–15 reps/
LEVEL-ONE EXERCISES, WEDNESDAY	**WORKOUT 1**	
Squat	1 set, 10–15 reps/	
Lunge	1 set, 10–15 reps/	
Calf raise	1 set, 10–15 reps/	
Crunch with a cross	1 set, 10–15 reps/	
Opposite arm and leg raise	1 set, 10–15 reps/	
LEVEL-TWO EXERCISES, MONDAY AND FRIDAY	**WORKOUT 1**	**WORKOUT 2**
Dumbbell fly	1 set, 10–15 reps/	1 set, 10–15 reps/
Dumbbell bench press	2 sets, 10–12, 8–10 reps/	2 sets, 10–12, 8–10 reps/
Lat pulldown to front	1 set, 10–15 reps/	1 set, 10–15 reps/
Bent-over dumbbell row	2 sets, 10–12, 8–10 reps/	2 sets, 10–12, 8–10 reps/
Lateral raise	1 set, 10–15 reps/	1 set, 10–15 reps/
Rotation press	2 sets, 10–12, 8–10 reps/	2 sets, 10–12, 8–10 reps/
LEVEL-TWO EXERCISES, WEDNESDAY	**WORKOUT 1**	
Squat	3 sets, 10–12, 8–10, 8–10 reps/	
Lunge	3 sets, 10–12, 8–10, 8–10 reps/	
Calf raise	3 sets, 10–12, 8–10, 8–10 reps/	
Crossover	1 set, 10–15 reps/	
Superman	1 set, 10–15 reps/	

mended number of sets and
repetitions. Track how many

sets and reps you actually
finish by recording those

numbers to the right sides of
the slashes.

WEEK 2

WORKOUT 1	WORKOUT 2
2 sets, 8–12 reps/	2 sets, 8–12 reps
2 sets, 8–12 reps/	2 sets, 8–12 reps
2 sets, 8–12 reps/	2 sets, 8–12 reps

WORKOUT 1

2 sets, 8–12 reps/

2 sets, 8–12 reps/

2 sets, 8–12 reps/

2 sets, 8–12 reps/

2 sets, 8–12 reps/

WORKOUT 1	WORKOUT 2
2 sets, 8–12 reps/	2 sets, 8–12 reps/
2 sets, 10–12, 8–10 reps/	2 sets, 10–12, 8–10 reps/
2 sets, 8–12 reps/	2 sets, 8–12 reps/
2 sets, 10–12, 8–10 reps/	2 sets, 10–12, 8–10 reps/
2 sets, 8–12 reps/	2 sets, 8–12 reps/
2 sets, 10–12, 8–10 reps/	2 sets, 10–12, 8–10 reps/

WORKOUT 1

3 sets, 10–12, 8–10, 8–10 reps/

3 sets, 10–12, 8–10, 8–10 reps/

3 sets, 10–12, 8–10, 8–10 reps/

2 sets, 8–12 reps/

2 sets, 8–12 reps/

(continued)

	WEEK 1	
LEVEL-THREE EXERCISES, MONDAY AND FRIDAY	**WORKOUT 1**	**WORKOUT 2**
Incline dumbbell press	1 set, 10–15 reps/	1 set, 10–15 reps/
Dumbbell fly	2 sets, 10–12, 8–10 reps/	2 sets, 10–12, 8–10 reps/
Dumbbell bench press	2 sets, 10–12, 8–10 reps/	2 sets, 10–12, 8–10 reps/
Reverse-grip pulldown	1 set, 10–15 reps/	1 set, 10–15 reps/
Lat pulldown to front	2 sets, 10–12, 8–10 reps/	2 sets, 10–12, 8–10 reps/
Bent-over dumbbell row	2 sets, 10–12, 8–10 reps/	2 sets, 10–12, 8–10 reps/
Bent-over lateral raise	1 set, 10–15 reps/	1 set, 10–15 reps/
Lateral raise	2 sets, 10–12, 8–10 reps/	2 sets, 10–12, 8–10 reps/
Rotation press	2 sets, 10–12, 8–10 reps/	2 sets, 10–12, 8–10 reps/
LEVEL-THREE EXERCISES, WEDNESDAY	**WORKOUT 1**	
Squat	3 sets, 10–12, 8–10, 6–8 reps/	
Lunge	3 sets, 10–12, 8–10, 6–8 reps/	
Calf raise	3 sets, 10–12, 8–10, 6–8 reps/	
Catch	3 set, 8–12 reps/	
Isometric back extension	3 sets, 4 reps (4-sec holds)/	

those tips are specific to the exercise they accompany, several apply to virtually all of the exercises you'll be doing:

■ Keep constant tension on the targeted muscle.
■ Do every motion slowly, and stay in control on the way down as well as up. Avoid bouncing, jerking, or "throwing" the weight, and don't let gravity or momentum do the work.

■ Pause and flex the targeted muscle at the top of the movement before returning to the starting position.
■ Don't rest or relax between reps.
■ Focus on feeling your chest, shoulder, or back muscles doing the work. Otherwise the arms tend to take over, defeating your purpose.
■ Keep your lower back in its natural position. If you have to arch or round or rock your back, you're probably using too

WEEK 2

WORKOUT 1	WORKOUT 2
2 sets, 8–12 reps/	2 sets, 8–12 reps/
2 sets, 10–12, 8–10 reps/	2 sets, 10–12, 8–10 reps/
2 sets, 10–12, 8–10 reps/	2 sets, 10–12, 8–10 reps/
2 sets, 8–12 reps/	2 sets, 8–12 reps/
2 sets, 10–12, 8–10 reps/	2 sets, 10–12, 8–10 reps/
2 sets, 10–12, 8–10 reps/	2 sets, 10–12, 8–10 reps/
2 sets, 8–12 reps/	2 sets, 8–12 reps/
2 sets, 10–12, 8–10 reps/	2 sets, 10–12, 8–10 reps/
2 sets, 10–12, 8–10 reps/	2 sets, 10–12, 8–10 reps/

WORKOUT 1

3 sets, 10–12, 8–10, 6–8 reps/

3 sets, 10–12, 8–10, 6–8 reps/

3 sets, 10–12, 8–10, 6–8 reps/

3 sets, 8–12, reps/

3 sets, 5 reps (4-sec holds)/

much weight or have already exhausted the targeted muscles.

■ Never hold your breath.

BEYOND THE EXERCISES

A troubleshooting section at each level addresses the frequently asked questions of beginning strength trainers. Each level also includes instructions for your cardiovascular program. Cardio effort can help or hurt when you're trying to build muscle; the "Aerobic Essentials" will show you the kind and amount of cardio work that will work best for your purposes.

Finally, you'll find simple nutrition tips in each of the next three chapters. Even the most serious strength training can be sabotaged by a sloppy diet, so I'll show you how to eat to energize your workouts, fuel your muscle growth, and lose the flab to uncover the V-shape waiting to emerge.

CHAPTER NINE

ESSENTIAL FOUNDATION
LEVEL ONE

Start the three focus exercises that form the foundation of your 6-week program: One emphasizes the chest, one the shoulders, and one the upper back. You'll also do five other exercises for all-around development and increased muscle-building testosterone.

- Do three upper-torso exercises twice a week.
- Do five midsection and lower-body exercises once a week.
- Begin a 3-day-a-week cardiovascular program.
- Review your diet and focus on protein.

THE LEVEL-ONE ROUTINE

- Do your chest, upper-back, and shoulder exercises on Monday and Friday. Do the other exercises on Wednesday.
- In Week 1, do one set of 10 to 15 repetitions for all the exercises. In Week 2, do two sets of 8 to 12 reps of all the exercises.
- Use a weight you can just manage to lift for the number of reps you plan to do. Use more weight each Friday than you did the previous Monday.
- During Week 2, do both sets of each exercise before moving on to the next.
- Rest 1 minute between sets and exercises.

BENEFITS
OF LEVEL ONE

Stronger chest, back, and shoulder muscles

Improved strength and flexibility from head to toe

Increased release of muscle-building hormones

More energy throughout the day

Bolstered self-confidence

Dumbbell Bench Press (Chest)

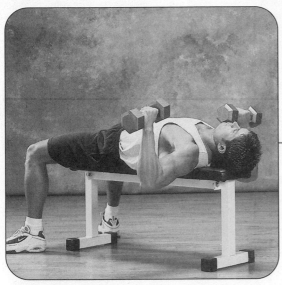

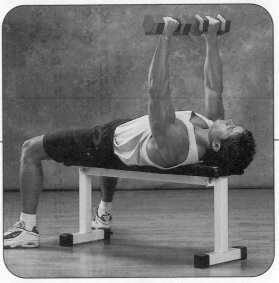

READY, SET:

Lie on your back on a bench, holding a pair of dumbbells just above and outside your chest. Your feet should be flat on the floor for stability, your legs slightly parted, and your back and head firm against the bench.

GO:

Push the weights up in a slanting motion so they almost meet when your arms are extended. Pause. Slowly lower them back to the starting position, pause and repeat.

PERFORMANCE TIPS

■ Make sure your head and shoulder blades stay pressed against the bench and your lower back maintains a natural arch throughout the movement. If you have to arch your lower back excessively to push the dumbbells up, you're using too much weight.

■ Don't clank the weights together at the top. That takes tension off your muscles.

■ Lower the weights as far as they want to go in your natural range of motion. If you stop them short of a full descent or try to lower them past your comfort zone, you risk strained shoulders and limited gains.

■ Lower and extend your arms without rotating your shoulders or turning your wrists. The dumbbells should be exactly perpendicular to your body at both ends of the movement.

Bent-Over Row (Upper Back)

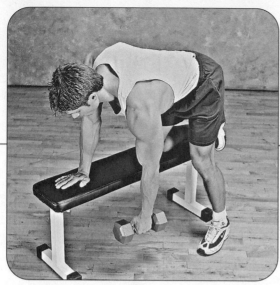 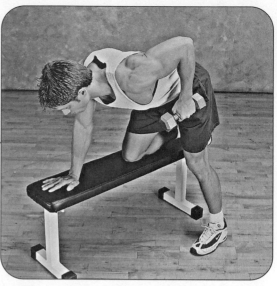

READY, SET:

Hold a dumbbell in one hand as you place your opposite hand and knee on a weight bench. Your back should be flat and parallel to the bench. Let your arm hang straight down from your shoulder as you grip the dumbbell with your palm facing in.

GO:

Pull the weight straight up toward the side of your abdomen, finishing with your elbow pointing toward the ceiling. Pause, then slowly lower the weight back to the starting position. Repeat. When you finish all your reps with one arm, hold the weight in your other hand, put your other knee and hand on the bench, and do the same number of reps.

PERFORMANCE TIPS

■ Do the prescribed number of reps with your non-dominant arm first. That is, if you're right-handed, do the exercise with the dumbbell in your left hand before switching over to your stronger right hand. Remember, it's not a set until you've done the same number of repetitions on each side.

■ Tighten your abs for stability and keep them that way.

■ Make sure you pause at the top and bottom of the movement, and that you stay in control as you lower the weight slowly. Momentum and gravity are your enemies here—the more you dominate them, the faster you'll build muscle.

Rotation Press (Shoulders)

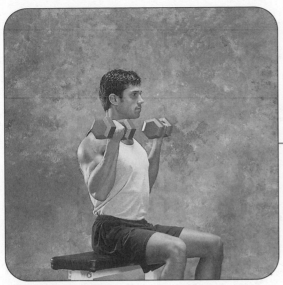 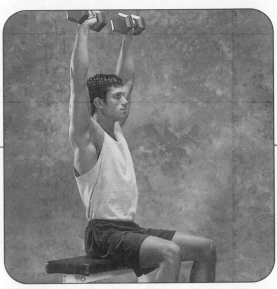

READY, SET:

Sit on the end of the bench and hold a pair of dumbbells underneath your chin with an underhand grip, the backs of your hands facing away from you. Pull your shoulders back, push your chest out, and look straight ahead. Set your feet flat on the floor, shoulder-width apart.

GO:

As you push the weights up directly over your head, rotate your hands so your palms face forward in an overhand grip when your arms are fully extended. Pause, then lower the weights, rotating your hands back to the starting position.

PERFORMANCE TIPS

- Keep your torso in the same position throughout the lift. Leaning back as you push the weights over your head is murder on your lower back and sacrifices results. If you can't help arching your back as you lift, you're probably holding too much weight.

- Don't touch the dumbbells together at the top. Your shoulders will work harder if you keep the weights apart.

- Extend your arms fully at the top of the movement, but don't lock your elbows. Bend them ever so slightly to keep tension on your shoulder muscles.

Squat (Thighs and Gluteals)

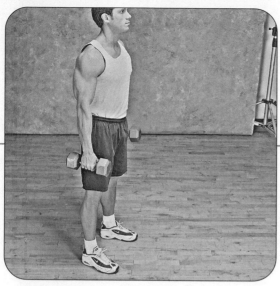
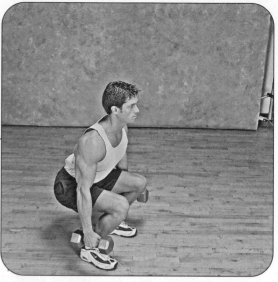

READY, SET:

Hold a pair of dumbbells, letting your arms hang straight down from your shoulders. Stand with your feet a little wider than shoulder-width apart, your toes pointed out slightly, and your knees unlocked. Pull your shoulders back, push your chest out, and look straight ahead. Your lower back should be in its naturally arched position, and your head should be in alignment with your spine.

GO:

Bend your knees to lower yourself, and as you sink, push your butt back as if you were sitting down in a chair. Go down slowly until your thighs are parallel to the floor or until your heels start to rise off the floor. Slowly rise back up to the starting position and repeat.

PERFORMANCE TIPS

■ If you're a newcomer to the squat, do the set without weights for your first workout. Hold your hands straight out from your shoulders.

■ With or without weights, keep your heels flat on the floor and your back in its natural alignment. That won't be easy at first.

■ It may take weeks or even months to be able to get down to where your thighs are parallel to the floor. Meanwhile, get as far down as you can without lifting your heels or leaning forward.

■ Always lower yourself slowly and never bounce back up.

Lunge (Thighs and Gluteals)

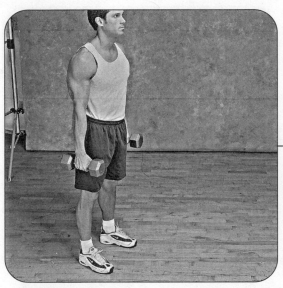
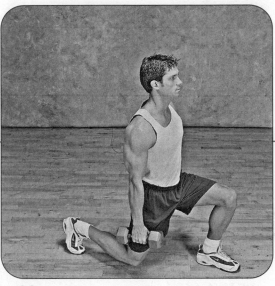

READY, SET:

Hold a pair of dumbbells and let your arms hang straight down from your shoulders. Stand with your feet a little wider than shoulder-width apart, your toes pointed out slightly, and your knees unlocked. Pull your shoulders back, push your chest out, and look straight ahead. Your lower back should be neither arched nor rounded, and your head should be in alignment with your spine.

GO:

Step one leg forward a little farther than you would in a normal stride, landing on your heel as you bend that knee as far as you can without letting it go ahead of your toes. At the same time, lower your other knee until it's just short of touching the floor behind you. Push back off your forward heel and return to the starting position.

PERFORMANCE TIPS

- Do this without weights for your first workout. When you can do 15 repetitions with each leg, add the dumbbells.
- Start with your nondominant leg, and alternate legs until you've done the prescribed number of reps on each. If you do all the reps with your stronger side first, you may not be able to finish the same number with your weaker side, increasing any strength discrepancy you might have.
- Never bounce the back knee off the ground.
- Keep your torso upright. Don't let it drift forward as you get tired.

Calf Raise (Lower Legs)

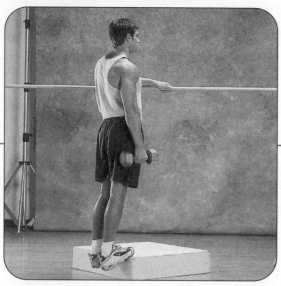

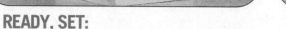

READY, SET:

Hold one dumbbell and let that arm hang straight down from your shoulder. Stand on the balls of your feet on a raised step or platform (a staircase works well) with your feet hip-width apart and your heels hanging off the step, as low as they'll go. Use your free hand to hold on to whatever you can for support, such as a banister.

GO:

Raise your heels as high as possible, distributing your weight toward your big toes. Pause, then slowly return to the starting position. Pause again. Repeat.

PERFORMANCE TIPS

- Each workout, alternate the hand in which you hold the weight. Or do half of the repetitions with the weight in one hand, then switch for the other half.

- Always go as high as you can and as low as you can on each repetition. You build the most muscle that way.

- Be sure to pause at both positions and move slowly. Bouncing up and down with the help of momentum and gravity isn't going to strengthen your calf muscles.

Crunch with a Cross (Abdominals)

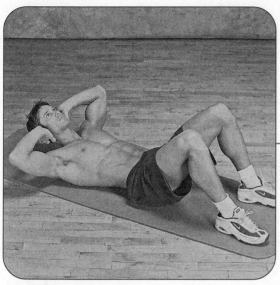

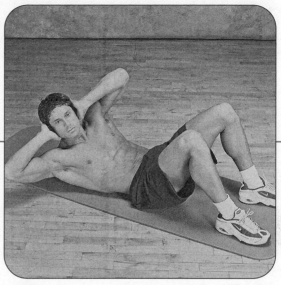

READY, SET:

Lie on your back with your knees bent, your feet flat on the floor, your head and neck relaxed, and your hands behind your ears.

GO:

Use the upper muscles of your abdomen to raise your rib cage toward your pelvis and lift your shoulder blades off the floor as you cross your right shoulder toward your left knee. Pause, then slowly lower back to the starting position. Repeat, this time crossing your left shoulder toward your right knee. That's one repetition.

PERFORMANCE TIPS

- Make sure your shoulder blades come off the floor each time. Don't just move your head and neck.
- Raise and lower yourself slowly. Don't use momentum or gravity to get through the repetitions.
- Remember to breathe. Beginners tend to hold their breath during any kind of crunch, which accomplishes nothing.
- Pause, but don't rest, at the bottom of the movement. Pause at the top of the movement, after you've exhaled, and feel the squeeze go deeper into your abdominal muscles.
- Keep your head and neck relaxed.

Opposite Arm and Leg Raise (Lower Back)

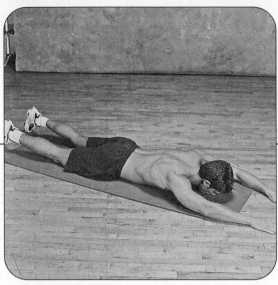 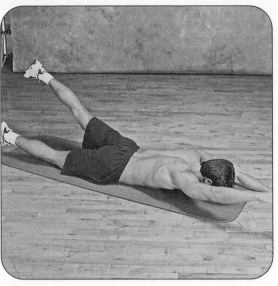

READY, SET:

Lie facedown on the floor with your arms and legs extended and your palms flat on the floor in front of you.

GO:

Simultaneously raise your right arm and left leg to a comfortable height. Hold for 2 seconds, then slowly lower to the starting position. As soon as your arm and leg lightly touch the floor, repeat with your left arm and right leg. Alternate until you've done all the recommended repetitions on each side.

PERFORMANCE TIPS

■ As you raise your arm and leg, also try to extend them by making them reach out farther.

■ As you raise your leg, you'll feel this exercise in your gluteals and hamstrings (back-thigh muscles) as well as your lower back.

■ For more of a challenge, keep your nonworking arm and leg off the floor throughout the exercise. That is, as you raise your right arm and left leg, keep your left arm and right leg slightly off the floor. Then don't let the raised limbs quite reach the floor as you lower them. Doing this on both sides for the whole set will keep more tension on your lower back.

CARDIO DAYS

Your goal is to do a half hour of aerobic exercise 3 days a week, 20 minutes of which should be brisk enough to get your heart beating at 65 percent to 85 percent of its estimated maximum rate—220 minus your age. You want to start with 5 minutes at a fairly easy pace, followed by the 20 minutes at your target heart rate, and finishing with 5 easy minutes.

If you're in good cardiovascular condition, start with this full routine and stick with it throughout the Core Program (with some variations at Levels Two and Three). If you've already been training aerobically, you may even have to reduce your workload.

Aerobic newcomers should work their way up to the ideal 5-20-5 cardiovascular routine described above. Aim for a 15-minute aerobic workout three times a week. Do 5 minutes at an easy pace, then 5 in your target heart-rate zone, and finish with 5 easy minutes.

How do you know your heart rate? The better cardio machines do the job for you, reading it as you grip a sensor. Otherwise, take your pulse. Put two fingers to your wrist or the side of your neck and count the throbs for 10 seconds. Multiply by six to get the per-minute rate.

Whether you're a beginner or a veteran, do the following.

- Take a day of rest between aerobic workouts.
- Do your aerobic work on days you don't strength train: Tuesday, Thursday, and Saturday.

- If you must lift and do cardio on the same day, do the weight exercises first. Muscles respond better when they're worked starting fresh, but previous lifting won't affect your aerobic performance much.
- Respect the 5-minute easy-pace segment before working in your target heart-rate zone. Your body needs that time to increase its core temperature, lubricate your joints, and adjust its chemistry.
- Same goes for the 5-minute cooldown at the end. Your heart needs to slow down gradually. A sudden stop can cause blood to pool in your extremities, which is dangerous.

PACK IN THE PROTEIN

As you get into the Core Program, it's time to start eating with your muscles in mind. At Level One, you have just three simple nutritional tasks.

- Ignore everything you've ever heard or read about diets, good foods, and bad foods.
- Start paying attention to what you're actually eating at each meal.
- Every day, aim for 7 to 9 grams of protein per 10 pounds of body weight.

Trying to make sense out of conflicting, one-size-fits-all dietary advice is frustrating and irrelevant to your strength-training goals. But taking time to really notice what you're eating—the proportion of carbohydrates to fat and protein, for example—will

■ I have no idea how much weight to use. What's a good average weight to start with for each exercise?

Even if there were such a thing as an average starting weight, it would still be a worthless number for you. You could be above or below average, even if you're a complete beginner. But you have three other things to go on—form, fatigue, and repetitions.

In the first week at this level, all the exercises have a minimum rep count of 10. Let that be your marker. The ideal weight will allow you to be able to complete the 10th rep, but no more.

The first time you do an ex-ercise, err on the light side in guessing how heavy a dumb-bell to use. Then, if you can do 10 reps too easily with it, se-lect a heavier dumbbell next time. If you exhaust the muscle before you get to 10, end the set and go lighter next time (which means delaying for the time being your goal of using more weight on Friday than on Monday).

If you haven't found the right weight after the second workout of the first week, continue the adjustments during the second week. Keep your rep count at 10 (which falls within the 8-to-12 range prescribed) until you find a good weight. When you can do 12 with it, increase the weight and aim for at least 8 repetitions with the heavier load.

■ It's hard to stay steady as I lift. The dumbbells don't go up together and they wobble all over the place.

Most guys start their weight training with one side stronger than the other. That's hardly surprising, since most activi-ties—tennis, bowling, brief-case carrying, channel surfing—emphasize your dom-inant arm. This discrepancy makes it hard to move dumb-bells at the same speed and with the same range of motion.

Don't try to compensate for the difference. Use the same weight in both dumbbells and

prepare you to make food choices that are good for your muscle development, not to mention your overall health.

Start out by keeping track of your pro-tein intake, which is usually measured in grams. At 7 to 9 grams per 10 pounds of body weight, a healthy and active 200-pound man who's training to build muscle mass should eat about 150 to 180 grams of protein a day, more than twice the absurdly low recommended daily al-lowance. Why so much? Your muscles use it to repair themselves after a workout, grow bigger, and then main-tain that size.

It's not hard at all to get that much daily protein. Emphasize fish and lean cuts of meat; for example, 8 ounces of very lean beef will get you 55 grams of protein. And use low-fat dairy products; they're not any lower in protein. Beans and nuts also offer protein.

concentrate on good form. Things will even out as you gain coordination.

Another thing: Your muscles move because nerve impulses from the brain tell them to. New movements require new neuromuscular relationships. Simply put, your muscles have to learn how to do the lift. Until they do, the movement will be jerky, and probably not very pretty.

The good news is that they learn fast. And with that newfound neuromuscular coordination comes quick strength gains—even before your muscles grow bigger. So the cure for the wobblies is to keep on lifting, focusing on form.

■ Why aren't there any specific exercises for my arms? Shouldn't I be working them along with legs in the Wednesday workout?

You're working them on Monday and Friday. Just about any lift featuring your chest, shoulders, or upper back is going to involve your arm muscles. At Level One, for example, the dumbbell bench press works your triceps as well as your pecs and delts. The bent-over row hits your biceps along with your lats and other back muscles. And you use your triceps in addition to your delts to do the rotation press. The way the Core Program is structured, you always have 3 or 4 days in between workouts for

your upper-body muscles—including your arms—to recover and grow bigger and stronger. If you added arm exercises on Wednesday, you'd end up working your arm muscles 3 days a week, with only 2 days to recover in between workouts. That isn't enough time for them to recover, and as a result of their exhaustion, you'd get worse results on your chest, shoulder, and back exercises.

You probably want to do arm-specific exercises when you finish with the Core Program to help them develop fully. But rest assured, they will grow bigger when you're challenging yourself with tough upper-torso exercises like presses, rows, and pulldowns.

Finally, a few words about protein shakes: They get lauded in some circles as the mother's milk of muscle-builders, demonized in others as a waste of money. The truth, of course, is somewhere in between. A whey-protein supplement can be added to a fruit smoothie to give you a solid pre- or post-workout meal. Meal-replacement powders (MetRx, Myoplex, Grow!) made with whey or casein protein, or a combination of the two, contain both protein and carbohydrates. Blend them with water to get about 40 grams of protein with just 300 or so calories.

These products don't have any magical qualities you won't find in real food—but they certainly rank high in convenience. And if you have to choose between a 300-calorie meal-replacement shake or a Snickers bar for a midafternoon snack, the choice is pretty obvious.

CHAPTER TEN

ESSENTIAL EXPANSION
LEVEL TWO

Now you're ready to expand your routine for bigger results.

- Three new upper-torso exercises—one each for your chest, shoulders, and upper back. That brings the total to six.
- Two new midsection exercises to add variety.
- Increased aerobic effort.
- The best protein-carbohydrate-fat ratio.

THE LEVEL-TWO ROUTINE

- Continue doing the chest, shoulder, and back exercises on Monday and Friday, and the other exercises on Wednesday.
- In the first week, do one set of each of the three new upper-torso exercises before you do two sets of the upper-torso exercises you learned at Level One.
- The second week, do two sets of the new upper-torso exercises and two sets of the held-over exercises.
- Do one set of all five midsection and lower-body exercises the first week, and two sets the second week.
- Use more weight on each Friday than the previous Monday.
- Rest 1 minute between exercises.

BENEFITS
OF LEVEL TWO

Noticeably increased upper-torso strength

Improved aerobic capacity

Flab loss from increased exercise

Better weight management from speeded-up metabolism, exercise, and diet adjustments

More energy from a higher fitness level and balanced diet

More overall strength

Dumbbell Fly (Chest)

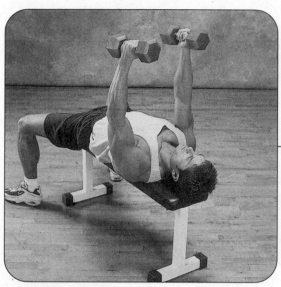 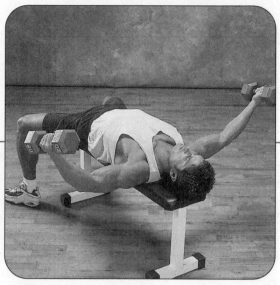

READY, SET:

Grab a pair of dumbbells and lie on your back on a flat bench with your feet planted on the floor. Hold the dumbbells over your chest with your palms facing each other, arms extended, and elbows slightly bent.

GO:

Slowly lower the dumbbells in arcing motions until your upper arms are parallel to the floor and your palms face the ceiling. Pause, then lift the dumbbells along the same arcs to the starting position.

PERFORMANCE TIPS

■ Maintain the same bend in your elbows throughout the motion. It should be 45 degrees at most. You see many guys bending their elbows to 90 degrees (or more) when they lower the weights, then straightening their arms on the way up. That's a different exercise (sort of a hybrid press/fly combination), and involves the triceps, which you want to keep out of this exercise.

■ The key to this movement is keeping your chest tensed throughout. The slower you move the weights—particularly as you lower them—the more you'll feel your chest working, and the more you'll get out of the exercise.

■ Don't bang the dumbbells together at the top. It takes tension off your chest muscles, and annoys the hell out of anyone else in the weight room.

■ Don't let your forearms rotate as you go down or up. The dumbbells should stay at the same angle throughout the motion.

Dumbbell Bench Press (Chest)

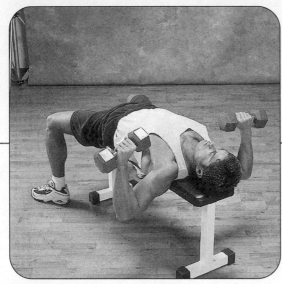
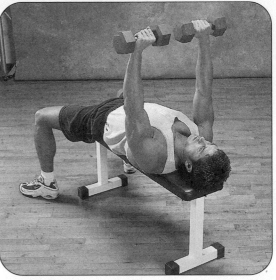

READY, SET:

As at Level One, use an overhand grip to hold two dumbbells just above and outside your chest as you lie back on a level bench. Your feet should be flat on the floor, and your back and head firm against the bench.

GO:

Perform the exercise as you did at Level One, but concentrate more on keeping your chest contracted throughout the motion. Push the weights up in a slanting motion so they almost meet when your arms are extended. Slowly lower back to the starting position, pause and repeat.

PERFORMANCE TIPS

■ Most guys perform chest exercises as strength movements—that is, they try to push as much weight as possible as fast as possible. But your goal in the Core Program is hypertrophy—making the muscles bigger. (You'll find strength routines in chapter 13.) That means keeping the muscles tensed throughout the exercise, not just during the lift. The following tips help you do that:

■ Don't lock your elbows when you extend your arms.

■ Don't clank the weights together at the top.

■ Lower and extend your arms without rotating your shoulders or turning your wrists. The dumbbells should be exactly perpendicular to your body at both ends of the movement.

Lat Pulldown to Front (Upper Back)

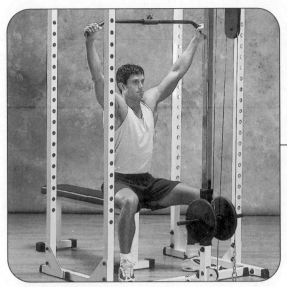
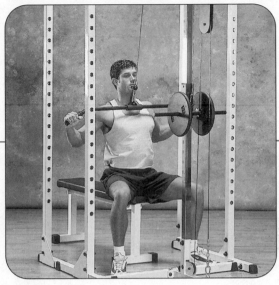

READY, SET:

Attach a long bar to a high cable pulley, and grab the bar with an overhand grip that's just beyond shoulder-width. Position yourself in front of the machine so you're facing the weight stack. Lean back slightly with your arms extended straight up.

GO:

Pull the bar down to your chest. Pause, then slowly return to the starting position.

PERFORMANCE TIPS

■ Don't rock back and forth as you perform the exercise. Hold your torso in one position as you pull the bar to your chest.

■ Bring the bar straight down, keeping your palms and wrists facing the cable in front of you. Don't rotate your shoulders.

■ Concentrate the effort on your upper back, rather than your biceps and forearms (which are also worked), by keeping your lats contracted and your hands and arms relaxed.

■ The angle at which you lean back can be anywhere between 15 and 45 degrees, and you can adjust it from set to set to emphasize different parts of your latissimus dorsi and trapezius. Just don't shift during the movement itself. That brings your lower back into the movement more than necessary.

Bent-Over Row (Upper Back)

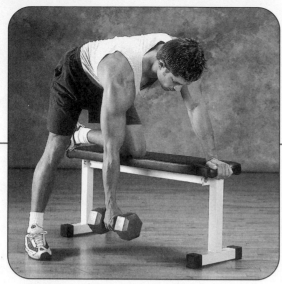 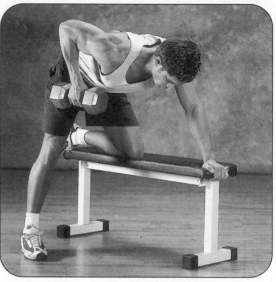

READY, SET:

Perform this exercise as you did at Level One, making an extra effort to focus on your upper-back muscles. Hold a dumbbell in one hand as you place your opposite hand and knee on a weight bench. Your back should be flat and parallel to the bench. Let your arm hang straight down from your shoulder as you grip the dumbbell with your palm facing in.

GO:

Think of your back muscles, not your arms, as the hardest workers as you pull the weight straight up toward the side of your abdomen, finishing with your elbow pointing toward the ceiling. Pause, then slowly lower the weight back to the starting position. Repeat. When you finish all your reps with one arm, do the same number of reps with the other.

PERFORMANCE TIPS

- Concentrate on the latissimus dorsi, the middle trapezius, and the rhomboids, as well as the posterior deltoid. Relaxing your hands and arms will help you focus the effort on your upper back.

- You can try a variation in which you hold your elbow away from your torso, involving more of the muscles across the top of your back—your rear deltoids, trapezius, and rhomboids—and less work from the lats. Some guys prefer this because it's more of a "feel" exercise. The lats are hard to feel on the regular dumbbell row, and many guys make it tougher by using weights that are too heavy, doing reps too fast, and adding torso movement that further disengages the lats.

- Keep your torso in one fixed position throughout the exercise.

Lateral Raise (Shoulders)

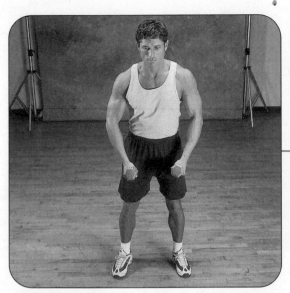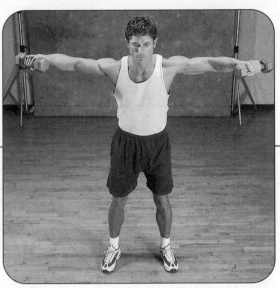

READY, SET:

Grab a pair of dumbbells and stand with your feet about hip-width apart, your knees slightly bent, your upper torso leaning forward slightly—your chin should be over your toes. Hold your arms straight down from your shoulders, with your palms facing each other and elbows slightly bent.

GO:

Lift the weights straight out to your sides until your upper arms are parallel to the floor and perpendicular to your torso. Pause, then slowly lower the dumbbells back to the starting position.

PERFORMANCE TIPS

- Your palms should face each other at the bottom of the movement and the floor at the top. Don't rotate your wrists or your shoulders.

- Flex your shoulders at the start of the movement. You should feel the dumbbells start to move upward as you do so. That shows you the deltoid muscles are engaged and taking charge of the lift.

- Maintain the same torso position throughout the lift. If you rock back and forth, you're using your hips and lower back to lift the weights, not your shoulders.

- Some guys prefer to do this exercise with one arm at a time. If you maintain good form, this variation can actually engage more muscles, since it's harder for your body to balance itself while lifting one weight at a time.

Rotation Press (Shoulders)

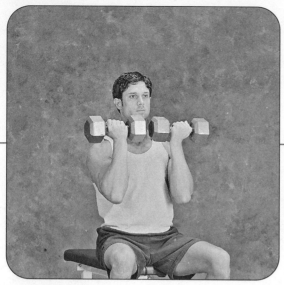 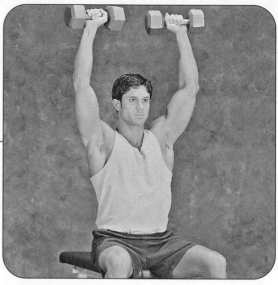

READY, SET:

Do the exercise as you did at Level One, but concentrate the effort even more on your shoulders so your deltoids work harder than your triceps. Hold a pair of dumbbells underneath your chin with an underhand grip, the backs of your hands facing away from you. Pull your shoulders back, push your chest out, and look straight ahead. Set your feet flat on the floor, shoulder-width apart.

GO:

As you push the weights up directly over your head, rotate your hands so your palms face forward when your arms are fully extended. Pause, then lower the weights, rotating your hands back to the starting position.

PERFORMANCE TIPS

■ You may prefer to do this exercise standing. That involves more muscles to keep your body balanced, but it ups the potential for cheating, too. Focus on keeping your entire body stable as you use your shoulders to lift the weights.

■ For another variation, raise the dumbbells at an angle away from your head so your arms make a V at full extension instead of an 11.

■ Whether you're sitting or standing, keep your torso in the same position throughout the lift. Don't lean back.

■ Remember not to lock your elbows at the top of the movement. Keep them slightly bent to maintain tension on your shoulder muscles.

Squat (Thighs and Gluteals)

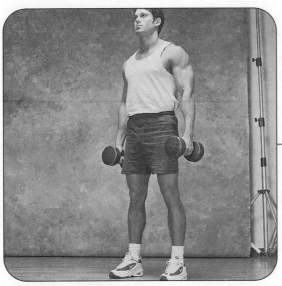

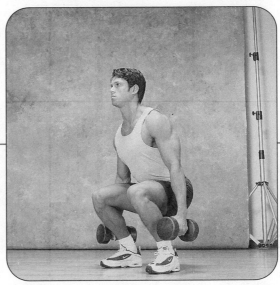

READY, SET:

If you performed this exercise without weights at Level One, add light dumbbells now. As you hold them, let your arms hang straight down from your shoulders. Stand with your feet a little wider than shoulder-width apart, your toes pointed slightly out, and your knees slightly bent. Pull your shoulders back, push your chest out, and look straight ahead. Your lower back should be in its naturally arched position, and your head should be in alignment with your spine.

GO:

Bend your knees to lower yourself, and as you sink, sit back as if you were sitting down in a chair. Go down slowly until your thighs are parallel to the floor. If you weren't able to get down that far at Level One, make it a point to try to descend a little lower this time. Slowly rise back up to the starting position and repeat.

PERFORMANCE TIPS

- Don't be discouraged if you still feel awkward doing squats. Your work will pay off in your gluteals, hamstrings, quadriceps, and lower back.

- If you have some experience with weights and have done squats before, you'll probably prefer the barbell squat. Hold a barbell across your shoulders, resting it behind your neck on the upper middle part of your trapezius. When you pull back your shoulder blades, this muscle contracts to form a nice shelf to rest the bar on. The rest of the exercise is the same.

- Keep your heels flat on the floor and your back in its natural alignment.

Lunge (Thighs and Gluteals)

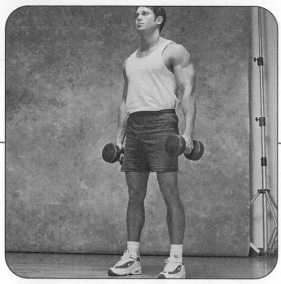
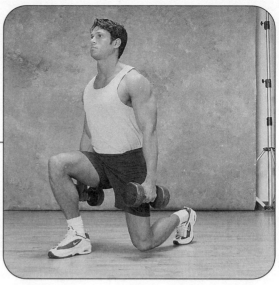

READY, SET:

If you didn't use any weights on this exercise at Level One and you can do 15 repetitions with each leg, start using dumbbells now. Hold them with your arms hanging straight down from your shoulders. Stand with your feet a little wider than shoulder-width apart, your toes pointed slightly out, and your knees slightly bent. Pull your shoulders back, push your chest out, and look straight ahead. Your lower back should be neither arched nor rounded, and your head should be in alignment with your spine.

GO:

Step one leg forward a little farther than you would in a normal stride, landing on your heel as you bend that knee 90 degrees. At the same time, lower your other knee until it's just short of touching the floor behind you. Push back off your forward heel to return to the starting position.

PERFORMANCE TIPS

- Lengthen your stride until you can bend your forward knee 90 degrees and still keep it behind your toes.
- If you're a fairly advanced lifter and trying to do lunges with heavier weights, you may be ready to move up to lunges with a barbell across your shoulders instead of dumbbells in your hands. The rest of the exercise is the same, although you have to work harder to keep your torso upright throughout the exercise.
- Never bounce the back knee off the ground.

Calf Raise (Lower Legs)

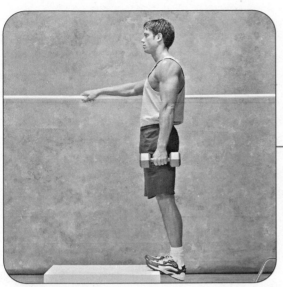 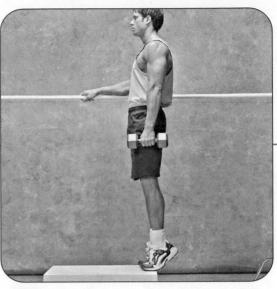

READY, SET:

Perform this exercise just as you did at Level One, adding more weight if you can. Hold a dumbbell and let your arm hang straight down from your shoulder. Stand on the balls of your feet on a raised step or platform (a staircase works well) with your feet hip-width apart and your heels hanging off the step, as low as they'll go. Use your free hand to hold on to whatever you can for support.

GO:

Raise your heels as high as possible, distributing your weight toward your big toes. Pause, then slowly return to the starting position. Pause again. Repeat.

PERFORMANCE TIPS

- Keep your legs mostly straight but with a very slight bend at the knee. That puts the calf muscles in their strongest position; they become considerably weaker if you lock your knees, which cuts off the top of the muscle from the exercise.

- You may prefer to work one calf at a time. Tuck the nonworking foot behind your working calf, and hold the weight on the side you're working. Don't forget to do the prescribed number of reps on each side.

- If you choose to continue working both calves at once, alternate the hand in which you hold the weight from workout to workout or set to set, or halfway through the reps.

Crossover (Abdominals)

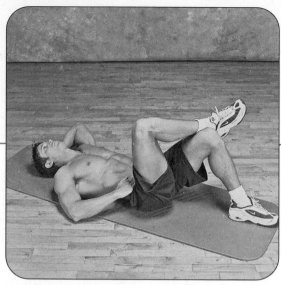 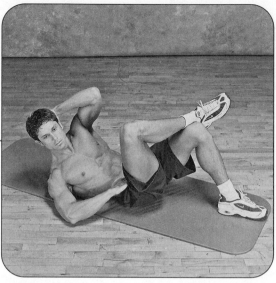

READY, SET:

Lie on your back with your knees up and your feet on the floor. Cross your left leg over your right leg. Your left ankle should rest just below your right knee, making a triangle between your legs. Put your right hand behind your head, with your elbow extended to the side. Place your left hand on your right obliques, or leave it at your left side. Rest your head on the floor.

GO:

Use your upper abdominals and right obliques to raise your right shoulder and cross it toward your left knee. Then slowly lower your shoulder back to the starting position. As soon as your shoulder blade lightly touches the floor, repeat. When you finish all your repetitions, switch positions and do the same number of repetitions crossing your left shoulder to your right knee.

PERFORMANCE TIPS

- Make sure your entire torso twists up and toward your knee. Don't just move your elbow or shoulder. Don't move your knee toward your shoulder.

- As you go up and across, feel the squeeze in your oblique muscles, which are more to the sides then the central abdominals. But you'll probably feel it in your upper abs, too, on the side you're working. That's fine.

- Don't rest at the bottom of the movement. Keep constant tension on your abs.

- Move up and down slowly, without using momentum to finish the repetitions.

Superman (Lower Back)

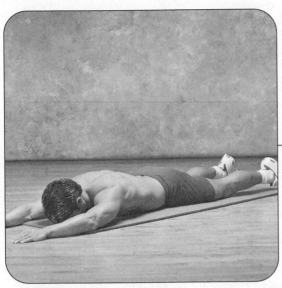

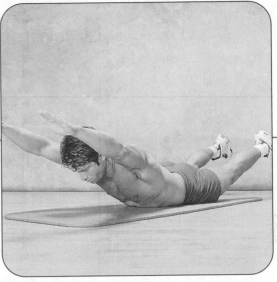

READY, SET:

Lie facedown on the floor with your arms stretched out above your head, your legs extended, and all four limbs angled out slightly. Your palms should face the floor.

GO:

Lift your arms and legs off the floor as if you were Superman flying. Hold for 3 seconds. Then slowly lower your arms and legs back to the starting position. As they lightly touch the floor, repeat.

PERFORMANCE TIPS

■ Your head and neck will also rise off the floor on this exercise, but don't allow your neck to hyperextend backward. Keep it in line with your shoulders throughout the exercise. However much your shoulders rise, that's how high your neck should lift.

■ As in the opposite arm and leg raise you performed at Level One, you'll feel a contraction in your gluteals and hamstrings as well as your lower back muscles.

■ If you can hold each contraction for longer than 3 seconds, do so. The more endurance you build in your lower back, the more improvement you'll feel in your posture.

■ How come the exercises from Level One seem harder now instead of easier?

Because at Level One you performed the three focus exercises with fresh muscles. Now each of those lifts is preceded by another one emphasizing the same primary muscle groups (chest, shoulders, or upper back). That makes them more challenging.

This is key to your progress. The Core Program is intentionally structured to emphasize three excellent focus exercises for each body part throughout the 6 weeks. By adding one new exercise for each body part at each new level, the program continually forces your muscles to work harder at the focus exercises.

■ Four weeks into the program and I'm doing only two exercises each for my chest, shoulders, and upper back. How can I make any progress at this rate?

By putting maximum effort into performing the two (soon to be three) prescribed exercises for each body part. You'll get the most benefit from hard work on a few top-drawer exercises, rather than spreading your effort throughout a marathon session of great, good, and mediocre exercises.

When you emphasize intensity over volume, you get the most out of your muscles when they're fresh, well-fueled, and prepared to do your bidding. The more volume you attempt—the more exercises and sets and repetitions you cram into a workout—the longer the workout becomes. Once a workout goes past the 1-hour mark, you risk putting your body into a catabolic, or muscle-depleting, state.

And, finally, the longer the workout, the more excuses you can come up with for skipping it. The Core Program is designed to get you in and out of the weight room as quickly as possible without sacrificing any potential benefits.

■ My shoulders are so weak I have to use embarrassingly light weights to do all the reps you ask. What's the matter with me?

Nothing. Light loads are the norm for a lot of shoulder exercises. In fact, beginners can be challenged without any weight in some shoulder exercises. The reason is simple: Your shoulder joint just wasn't designed to lift much weight in some positions.

Let's look at the lateral raise, for example. If you're a beginner, you may be surprised at how a piddling little poundage can turn into a challenge around the 10th or 12th repetitions. Any weight that exhausts your muscle at the end of a set is efficient, not embarrassing.

AEROBIC ESSENTIALS:
MOVING ON UP

If you were doing the 15-minute beginning aerobic routine at Level One, it's time to move a few steps closer to the ideal cardio workout for strength-trainers. During the first week at this level, do a 24-minute aerobic workout on 3 nonconsecutive days, broken down as follows:

- 5 minutes at an easy pace
- 6 minutes at your target pace
- 2 minutes at an easy pace
- 6 minutes at your target pace
- 5 minutes at an easy pace

Increase your cardio time to 28 minutes on each of your 3 aerobic days in the second week, as follows.

- 5 minutes at an easy pace
- 8 minutes at your target pace
- 2 minutes at an easy pace
- 8 minutes at your target pace
- 5 minutes at an easy pace

ADVANCED VARIATION

If you're already doing the full 30-minute workout—20 minutes of target-rate effort sandwiched by a 5-minute warmup and 5-minute cooldown—stay at that regimen. Your upper-torso work won't benefit from more or longer aerobic workouts.

But you can crank up the intensity once a week. In one of your 3 weekly cardio sessions, do some interval training. Start with the usual 5-minute warmup and then work as follows:

- 30 seconds at a hard pace—less than an all-out sprint but as much as you can keep up for half a minute.
- 1 minute at an easy pace
- Repeat that hard-easy sequence 8 to 12 times.

Your cooldown at the end can be for 4 minutes instead of 5, since it immediately follows the last 1-minute easy segment. Depending on how many times you repeat the hard-easy pairing, your interval workout will last from 21 to 27 minutes.

High-end cardio machines offer an advantage here, since you can control your intensity level at the push of a button while your heart rate is automatically monitored. But you can do interval training with any "natural" form of aerobic exercise such as running, biking, skating, skiing, or swimming faster and slower as you enjoy the outdoor scenery. (A lot of guys insist, though, that the most scenic cardio workout is in the aerobics-dance studio.)

EATING ESSENTIALS:
GETTING BALANCED

Since Level One, you've been making it a priority to consume 7 to 9 grams of protein a day per 10 pounds of body weight. Even though that's more than twice what's usually recommended for non-training men, you've probably discovered that it doesn't take much of a meal adjustment to get that much.

Now it's time to put your protein intake into context with the other two macronutrients: carbohydrates and fat. Generally speaking, the best diet for your goal of adding muscle mass to your upper body would consist of 20 percent of total calories from protein, 30 percent from fat, and 50 percent from carbohydrates.

Yes, there are diet doctors who advocate eating more protein calories than carbohydrate calories. And plenty of nutritionists insist that protein should be no more than 10 to 15 percent of your calories, and carbohydrates no less than 65 percent. Continue to observe your other nutrition priority from Level One—which is to tune out the contradictory information overload.

CARBOHYDRATES

These days, carbohydrates are either sanctified by those who think you should eat almost nothing else or vilified by adherents to Atkins and *Protein Power*-type diets, who'd ban the stuff if they could. But for your strength-training goals, 50 percent of total calories from carbohydrates should feel about right. That gives you enough energy to get through your workouts and helps you refuel your muscles post-exercise.

However, not all carbohydrates are worthy of space on your dinner plate. Go mostly with the slower-burning carbohydrates—that is, just about all vegetables, whole grain breads and cereals, beans, and fruits. Stay away from highly processed carbs, like white bread, white rice, low-fiber breakfast cereals, or anything made with enriched flour.

The other foods to stay away from are those in which the main ingredient is high-fructose corn syrup. Use of this sweetener has skyrocketed in the United States in the past 3 decades, along with the size of Americans' waistlines. It's found in sodas and fruit juices, along with some of the highly processed foods we've already warned you about. These foods are not only bad for your physique, they cause quick spikes and drops in your energy levels, which plays havoc with your moods and productivity, too.

FAT

Dietary fat has a way of turning into body fat because it's more than twice as calorie-rich as protein or carbohydrates. On the other hand, if you ate no fat at all, you'd probably turn into David Wells without the fastball, because you'd be hungry all the time. Truth is, you need fat, to the tune of about 30 percent of your total calorie intake.

Why? Because fat regulates your body temperature, protects your internal organs, provides cell-protecting vitamin E, helps regulate your testosterone production, and supplements the carb-produced energy. And, as mentioned, it satisfies your hunger.

But just as with carbohydrates, eating the right kind of fat makes the difference between a muscle-friendly and a muscle-hiding diet. As you learned at Level One, saturated fat from animal products like butter and red meat is associated with artery-clogging shifts in cholesterol levels. (Saturated fat is found in a few vegetable products, such as palm kernel oil.) Most nutritionists now recommend limiting saturated fat to 10 percent of your total daily calories. That would mean one-third of your daily fat intake on the diet that I recommend.

Trans fatty acids, or hydrogenated fats, are even worse. These are vegetable oils that have been chemically altered so margarine can feel like butter and packaged pies, cookies, and muffins can taste good. My advice: Avoid it altogether.

Instead, go for the unsaturated fats, especially the monounsaturated fats. These are the predominant fats in olives and olive oil, canola oil, peanuts and peanut butter, nuts and seeds, wheat germ, and avocados. (Foods contain a mix of fats, rather than 100 percent of one type.) Monounsaturated fats raise your levels of the heart-friendly form of cholesterol called high-density lipoprotein (HDL), while reducing the harmful low-density lipoprotein (LDL).

The other type of unsaturated fats, polyunsaturated, are a mixed bag. The omega-3 fats found in fish (salmon, tuna, mackerel) and flaxseeds are considered the healthiest for your heart, since they lower the most dangerous form of cholesterol.

On the other hand, omega-6 polyunsaturated fats—found in the greatest quantities in vegetable oils—are considered less beneficial.

REACHING THE RATIO

Putting all these pieces together into a diet that aids and abets your strength training may take a good deal of label reading and nutrition-chart consulting. Once you get a feel for that 50-30-20 carb-fat-protein ratio, though, the muscle-building meals will practically make themselves. Here, for example, is a sample dinner that's in the ballpark: poached salmon with a baked potato (low-fat sour cream, no butter); zucchini and garlic sauteed in olive oil; black beans; and a tossed green salad with olive-oil-based dressing.

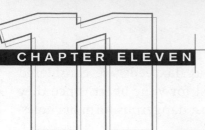
ESSENTIAL SUCCESS
LEVEL THREE

Here's where you make the transition from beginner to achiever.

- One new lift each for your chest, upper back, and shoulders.
- A new pair of midsection exercises to go with the three familiar lower-body exercises.
- The ideal aerobic workout for strength trainers, plus high-intensity variations.
- Eat energizing preworkout meals and recovery-enhancing postworkout meals.

THE LEVEL-THREE ROUTINE

- Continue doing the chest, back, and shoulder routines on Monday and Friday, and the lower-body and midsection exercises on Wednesday.
- Do one set of the new chest, upper-back, and shoulder exercises the first week, and two sets the second week.
- Do two sets each of the holdover upper-torso exercises.
- Do three sets each of the three lower-body exercises.
- Do three sets of the new abdominal exercise.
- Do three four-rep sets of the isometric back extension the first week, and three five-rep sets the second.
- Rest 30 to 60 seconds between sets and exercises.

BENEFITS
OF LEVEL THREE

A tremendous muscle-building stimulus for your chest, upper back, and shoulders

The emergence of noticeable muscle mass and the beginnings of a V-shaped torso

Increased efficiency of your heart and lungs from a steady aerobic program

Accelerated fat loss from a higher volume of exercise

A sense of accomplishment and a readiness for bigger gains

Incline Dumbbell Press (Chest)

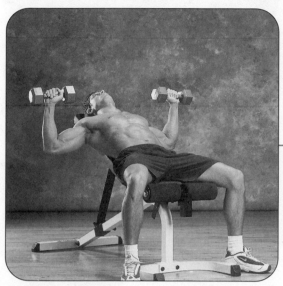

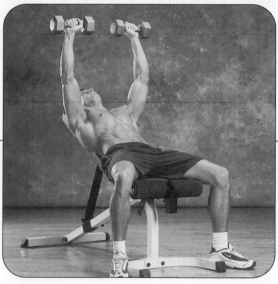

READY, SET:

Grab two dumbbells and lie back on an incline bench with your feet firmly on the floor or footrest and your head and shoulder blades planted against the inclined portion of the bench. Hold the dumbbells just outside your shoulders with your palms toward the ceiling.

GO:

Push the weights up in a slanting motion so they almost meet as your arms are fully extended. Pause and lower them slowly to the starting position.

PERFORMANCE TIPS

- The incline of the bench shifts more of the workload to the upper portion of your pectoralis major. The greater the incline, the less help you get from other portions of your chest. Between 30 and 45 degrees of incline is probably the best angle. Past 45 degrees, you start shifting the work to your front deltoids.

- Keep your chest tight throughout the motion. Imagine your chest pushing the dumbbells up, not your triceps or shoulders (though, of course, they're doing their share).

- As with the flat-bench dumbbell chest press, keep your feet planted flat, the back of your head touching the bench, and your shoulder blades pulled together in back. Don't arch your back excessively.

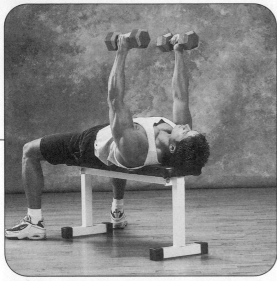 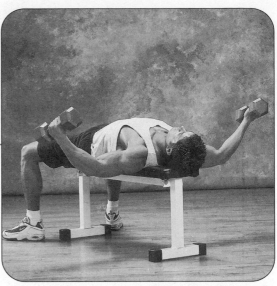

DUMBBELL FLY: Lying back, lower two dumbbells from an arms-extended position above your chest out to your sides. Return along the same arc.

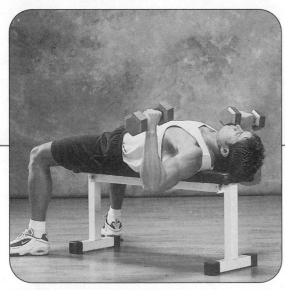 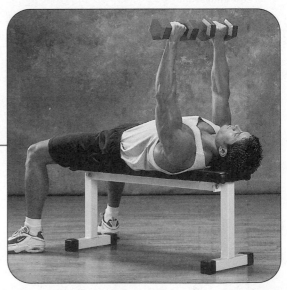

DUMBBELL BENCH PRESS: Lie back on a bench and push two dumbbells straight up from either side of your chest until your arms are extended.

▲ *If you need a refresher on the specific instructions for these exercises, see pages 63 and 64.*

Reverse-Grip Pulldown (Back)

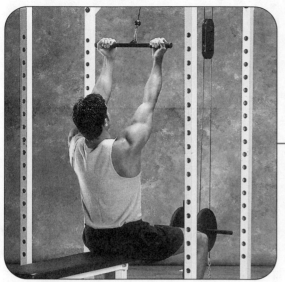 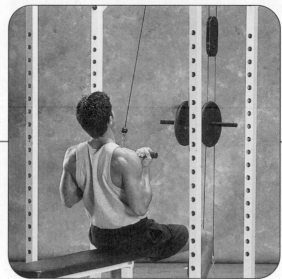

READY, SET:

Grab the lat-pulldown bar with an underhand grip, your hands just less than shoulder-width apart. Position yourself in front of the weight stack with your arms extended and elbows slightly bent. Lean back slightly.

GO:

Pull the bar down to the middle of your chest, bringing your elbows back as far as you can. Pause and slowly return to the starting position.

PERFORMANCE TIPS

■ Like the wide-grip pulldown, this exercise focuses on your latissimus dorsi. But the narrower, underhand grip brings other muscles into play, primarily your biceps as well as your chest. Still, you want your back to start the motion. So try to get the bar moving without any action from your arms—simply pull your shoulder blades together and down in back until the weight stack starts to move. Then finish the movement the normal way.

■ The weight plates you're using shouldn't rest on the weight stack when your arms are extended. Keep your lats contracted at the up position and don't rest between repetitions.

■ As with the wide-grip lat pulldown, keep your upper body steady as you lower the bar. If you have to rock or lift yourself up to get the bar down, you're using too much weight.

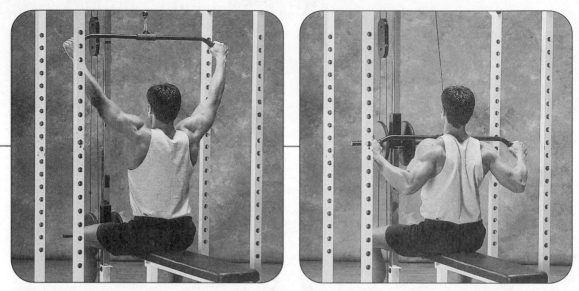

LAT PULLDOWN TO FRONT: Using a wide, overhand grip, bring the pulldown bar to your chest.

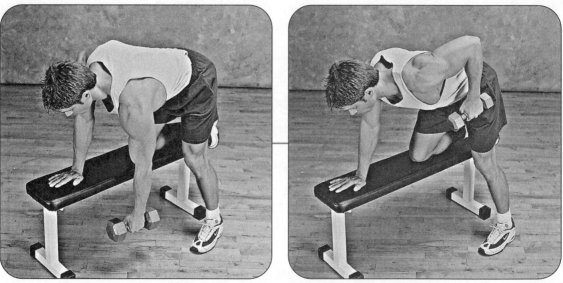

BENT-OVER ROW: From a bent-over position with your hand and knee on a weight bench, pull a dumbbell straight up to your side.

▲ *If you need a refresher on the specific instructions for these exercises, see pages 65 and 66.*

Bent-Over Lateral Raise (Shoulders)

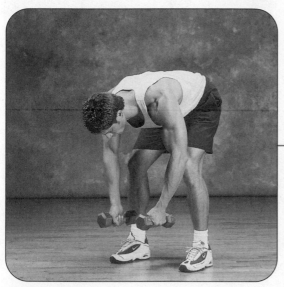

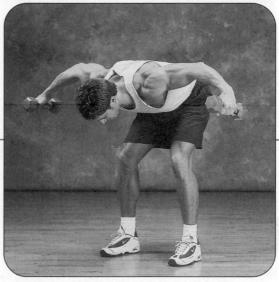

READY, SET:

Grab two dumbbells and stand with your feet slightly more than shoulder-width apart, your knees bent slightly. Bend over at the hips, holding the dumbbells in front of you with your arms hanging straight down, palms facing each other, and elbows bent slightly. The dumbbells should be an inch or two apart.

GO:

Raise the dumbbells up and out toward your side, until your upper arms are parallel to the floor. Pause, and then lower the dumbbells slowly to the starting position.

PERFORMANCE TIPS

■ The bent-over position moves the emphasis to the back of your deltoids, with some work taken on by your middle-back muscles. Bend forward at least 60 degrees and aim for 90 degrees—that is, your back parallel to the floor.

■ Keep a slight bend in your elbows and knees to protect your elbows and lower back from unnecessary stress. But don't straighten either set of joints. Moving your lower body takes work away from your shoulders, while straightening your arms turns this into a mediocre triceps exercise.

■ For comfort or variety, rest your forehead on the edge of a high bench. Or work one arm at a time, placing the other on a bench to support your body. Finally, you can bend forward and do the raises while seated at the edge of a bench, with the dumbbells hanging behind your knees at the starting position.

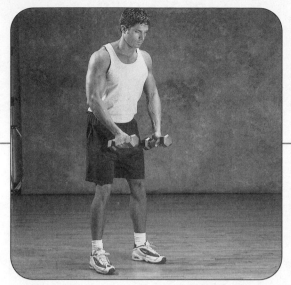 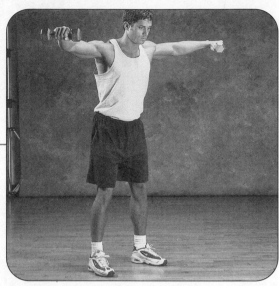

LATERAL RAISE: Raise two dumbbells laterally away from your sides until your body makes a T.

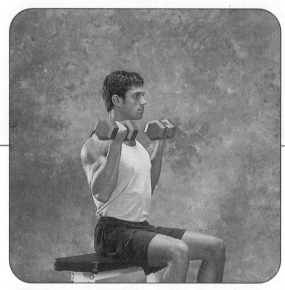 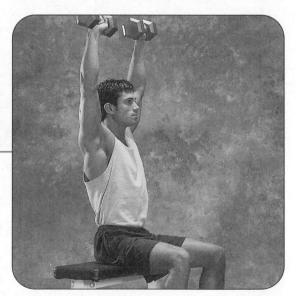

ROTATION PRESS: Push a pair of dumbbells from under your chin straight up over your head, rotating your grip from palms-in to palms-out.

▲ *If you need a refresher on the specific instructions for these exercises, see pages 67 and 68.*

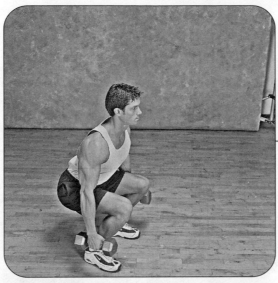

SQUAT: Holding dumbbells at your sides, lower yourself from a standing position as though you were taking a seat.

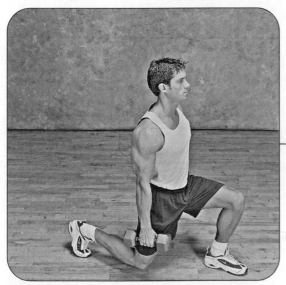

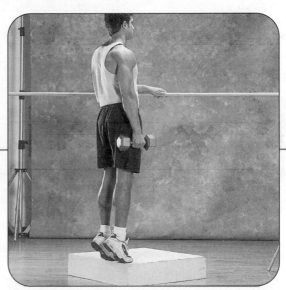

LUNGE: Holding dumbbells at your sides, step forward with one leg, bending that knee 90 degrees and lowering the other close to the floor.

CALF RAISE: Holding a dumbbell, stand with the balls of your feet on an elevated step and raise your heels from as low as they can go to as high as they can go.

▲ *If you need a refresher on the specific instructions for these exercises, see pages 54, 55, and 56.*

Catch (Abdominals)

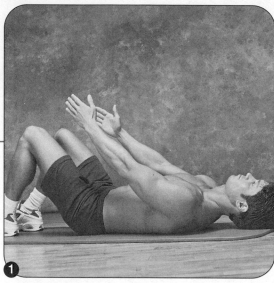

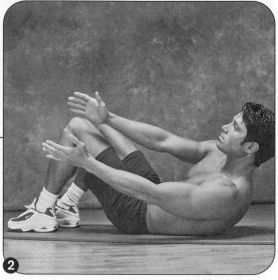

READY, SET:

Lie on your back with your knees bent, your feet flat on the floor, and your hands extended toward your knees.

GO:

Use your abdominal muscles to raise your torso on a diagonal line, lifting your right shoulder toward your left knee and reaching both hands above and to the outside of your left knee as if preparing to catch a beach ball. Hold for a second. Then slowly lower your shoulder back to the starting position, staying in control all the way down. As soon as your shoulder blade brushes the floor, start the same movement to your right side, lifting your left shoulder toward your right knee. That's one repetition.

PERFORMANCE TIPS

■ You may feel discomfort in your neck because your head is unsupported. If needed, support your head with one hand and reach with the other hand (making a one-handed catch).

■ Because you're moving your torso at a different angle, the contraction in your abdominals should feel different than it did during the crunch with a cross and the crossover that you performed at Levels One and Two. That's key to your ab development—different angles, different contractions.

Isometric Back Extension (Lower Back)

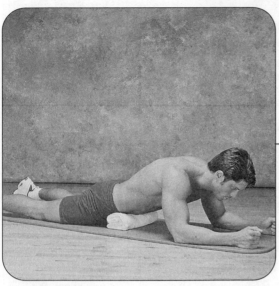 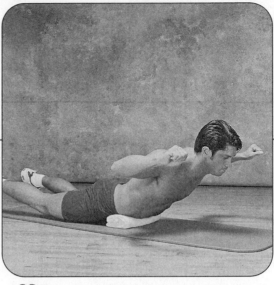

READY, SET:

Lie facedown on the floor with a rolled-up towel beneath your navel and your legs about shoulder-width apart. Lift your torso and rest your weight on your forearms, as if you were lying on the floor with a newspaper spread out in front of you.

GO:

Slowly lift your forearms off the floor and out to your sides while keeping your elbows flexed and your torso in the same position. Hold at this position for 4 or 5 seconds. Then, in a controlled motion, slowly lower your forearms back to the floor. Let some of the tension release from your lower back, and repeat.

PERFORMANCE TIPS

- Hold at the up position for 4 seconds the first week and 5 the second.

- Make sure you keep your torso and neck in the same position throughout the exercise.

- Breathe normally. Use your breath to count the 4- or 5-second hold at the elbows-up position—one strong breath per second.

- If you have a strong lower back, you may need to hold for longer than the 4 or 5 seconds prescribed to feel the exercise do its work.

■ How come I'm doing all these exercises with dumbbells? Why can't I use a barbell?

Barbells are great and you'll use them after the Core Program—except, of course, for those lifts like the rotation press that can't be done with barbells. But dumbbells have some advantages for a beginner or intermediate lifter.

First is the broader range of motion. Take the flat bench press: A barbell stops at your chest, while dumbbells go down a little lower than that. That's more work for your chest muscles.

Another advantage is that the independent movement of each arm helps you overcome any strength discrepancies. Just about anybody will be stronger on his dominant side when he starts lifting. Dumbbells help the two limbs grow equally strong.

Finally, your body uses more of its stabilizing muscles for balance and coordination when your two limbs are working independently of each other, rather than teaming up to move a single object. That leads to more complete muscular development.

■ I'm sick of lowering the weights so slowly. Wouldn't I build muscle faster if I lifted faster, using heavier weights? I know I'd enjoy it more.

You won't build more muscle lifting fast, because you'll finish the set with your muscles having spent little time under tension. You will, however, develop a neural system that's good at moving heavier weights. That's an important part of the training process, but the focus of the Core Program is on hypertrophy—making those muscles as big as possible in 6 weeks. Different goals, different methods.

Lifting the weights slower is also safer, since you're in full control of the load. That doesn't mean you'll get hurt if you lift heavier weights faster, but the risk is greater.

Finally, the slow descent ensures that your muscles work through a full range of motion, which helps maintain or even increase your flexibility. When you stay in control and resist gravity on the way down, you're using the same muscles you used on the way up.

■ The new exercises at Level Three are just variations on the ones I was already doing. Wouldn't something different be of better use?

It's essential to pay attention to details like grip and position when lifting weights. The variations offered by the new exercises at this level work different parts of your pecs, lats, and delts than the other versions. By inclining the bench for your presses, you shift the burden from your middle and lower chest to your upper pectorals. By bending over for the lateral raises, you make the posterior delts take over from the middle delts. Reversing and narrowing the grip on the pulldown makes your upper- and middle-back muscles work in different ways. So don't think of them as variations; they're different exercises.

It's natural to want totally new challenges. In fact, it's essential for continued progress. That's why the next section of the book (you're almost there!) introduces advanced routines and long-range strategies for constant variety.

AEROBIC ESSENTIALS:
GETTING IT DONE

If you've been working your way up to the prescribed thrice-weekly 30-minute aerobic session, you should reach your goal at this level. In the first week, you'll include the all-important 20 minutes at your target heart-rate level (a per-minute pulse of 65 to 85 percent of 220-minus-your-age). But it will be split into two 10-minute segments with an extra 2-minute easy-pace segment between them, as follows.

- A 5-minute warmup at an easy pace
- 10 minutes at your target pace
- 2 minutes at an easy pace
- 10 minutes at your target pace
- A 5-minute cooldown at an easy pace

In the second week, drop the extra 2-minute segment and do all 20 minutes of target-zone aerobic training consecutively, so your sessions look like this:

- A 5-minute warmup at an easy pace
- 20 minutes at your target pace
- A 5-minute cooldown

You're now performing the optimum aerobic workout for combining cardiovascular health with strength-training gains. Keep it up for 3 days a week as you go beyond the Core Program. When you're ready to go harder, blend in the following interval and sprint variations.

THE ADVANCED PLAN

You've been doing three-a-week aerobic workouts to pump up your cardiovascular system for a leaner and meaner muscle machine. But to repeat, too much emphasis on aerobics will actually hamper your strength-training goals. That's why it would be counterproductive to do more than the half-hour of cardiovascular work you've been doing up to now.

So how do you progress? By incorporating sprints into one of your aerobic sessions. A sprint is the anaerobic version of whatever aerobic activity you're doing, so it has something in common with lifting a weight in the way your muscles generate energy.

If you run (or bike, skate, swim, and so on) at a pace you can sustain for more than 2 minutes, you're using your aerobic ("with oxygen") energy system. If you run as hard as you can for 10 seconds, you're using creatine phosphate to power your movements. The CP system is one of your two anaerobic ("without oxygen") energy systems. The other is the lactic-acid system, which you can recognize by the familiar burning sensation within your muscles.

The following sprint routine also includes aerobic benefits, since you'll be moving continuously between the sprints. So it bridges the gap between your anaerobic weight-training workouts and your pure aerobic sessions. Substitute it on your first aerobic day of the week.

Start with a 5-minute warmup. Then:

- Go 10 seconds at a sprint pace—as hard as you can go
- 2 minutes at an easy pace
- Repeat the preceding hard-easy sequence until you've done 10 sprints

- 3 minutes at an easy pace added to the last 2-minute easy-pace segment, creating a 5-minute cooldown

On your second aerobic day, do the usual cardiovascular routine of 20 minutes at your target heart rate preceded and followed by 5 minutes at an easier pace.

On the final aerobic day, do the interval routine introduced at Level Two. Start with a 5-minute warmup. Then:

- 30 seconds at a hard pace—less than an all-out sprint but as much as you can keep up for half a minute.
- 1 minute at an easy pace
- Repeat that hard-easy sequence 8 to 12 times.
- 4 more minutes at an easy pace after the last 1-minute easy segment.

EATING ESSENTIALS:
POWER MEALS

At Levels One and Two, you began to shift your eating habits from what may have been an any-old-thing-that-tastes-good mode to a more balanced diet geared to adding muscle mass and subtracting body fat. Your focus has been on eating the right amount (and the right kind) of protein, carbohydrates, and fat.

Now move from the big picture to the small picture by planning pre- and post-workout meals that maximize your muscle gains. Your overall 50-30-20 ratio of carbs, fat, and protein won't change, of course, but you'll distribute those macronutrients in such a way that you'll feel

more energy during your workout and recover faster after it.

PREWORKOUT

For energized strength-training sessions, follow these guidelines.

- Eat an hour or two before your workout. If you must eat closer to the workout, make it a very small snack.
- Use less than the usual amount of fat in your preworkout meal. Fat digests slowly.
- Avoid sweets and processed foods. They turn on the insulin faucet full-blast, triggering a short-lived energy rush followed by an energy crisis—probably right when you're ready to hit the weights.
- Help yourself to the metered energy release of slower-burning carbohydrates, such as pasta and whole grains.
- Beware high-fiber foods such as vegetables, fruit, and bran cereals if you're within an hour of your workout. They're great foods in general, but are slow to digest. Eat them too soon before you train and you could experience some discomfort. (And if you don't, the other people in the weight room might.)
- Get some protein before your workout. Red meat isn't a great idea, however, since it's slow to digest. Instead, go for low-fat dairy

products (unless you're lactose-intolerant), eggs, or even whey-protein supplements. Those are all fairly easy on your stomach.

A liquid meal is a good option 2 hours before a workout. A simple smoothie made from fruit and fat-free yogurt with some wheat germ or low-fat granola thrown in will do the trick nicely.

POSTWORKOUT

After a hard workout, you want to help your muscles refuel and repair themselves as fast as possible. That makes your eating strategy a little different from your pre-workout routine:

- Get some fast-acting carbohydrates into you within a half-hour of the end of your workout. You want your body to release insulin to speed nutrients to your muscles. Bread and rice will work.
- Surprisingly, protein is not a high priority at this time. Sure, your muscles need protein to rebuild, but they get it from your overall supply, not necessarily from what you eat right after a workout. Five to 10 grams is enough. You can get that from a carton of yogurt, cup of milk, or an egg.
- On the other hand, more protein doesn't hurt anything. So if you're trying to divide your daily protein evenly across five or six meals, you can eat more protein in your first postworkout meal. It won't help you build more muscle in the postworkout hours, but your body will use it as it uses the rest of the protein you eat throughout the day. In other words, it's not wasted and won't slow your recovery.
- A liquid meal now and a bigger, well-balanced meal 2 hours later is an excellent postworkout strategy. Make yourself a flavored (nonfat) yogurt shake with plenty of fruit in it.

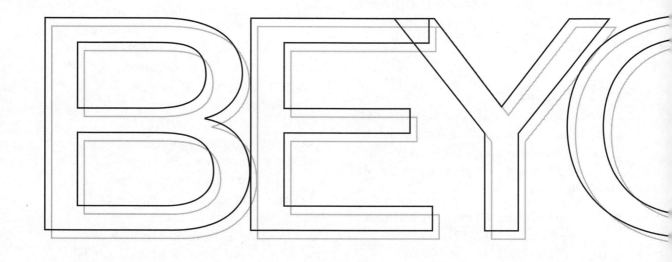

OND
THE CORE
PROGRAM

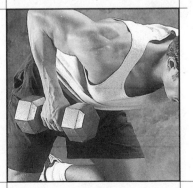

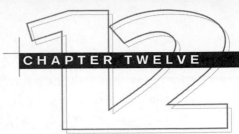

CHAPTER TWELVE

ESSENTIAL MAINTENANCE

Six weeks have come and gone since you first grabbed a pair of dumbbells to tackle the Core Program. Now you've aced the last set. Time to celebrate by taking a good look in the mirror. Notice anything?

Maybe what you notice is you need a bigger mirror. Your lats have grown enough to reshape your torso. Your middle delts have popped up into a couple of exclamation points on your emerging V-shape. Your chest has expanded and screams "hard muscle" instead of "instant pudding."

If so, great. More likely, though, the improvements are subtler. After all, you may not have noticed any significant changes in muscle size until after the fourth week. Still, your ratio of muscle mass to body fat has surely improved. Depending on your diet and previous exercise experience, you may have even lost a few pounds.

You sleep sounder at night from the increased activity. You're more energetic all day long from your exercise and sound eating habits. Improvements in strength and flexibility have put a spring in your step. You're enjoying these developments so much that you may not have even noticed how much better you feel about yourself.

Now what? Here's what you need to do to keep the results—and good feelings—coming.

UPPER-TORSO EXERCISE

The great thing about a 6-week program emphasizing your upper torso is that it leaves you eager to keep the gains coming. These are big muscles, and most guys will find that they grow fast once you get them started. If 6 weeks won't exactly turn you into George of the Jungle, it's enough to make you thirsty for more.

But whether you want to move forward or just hold on to what you built during the Core Program, you have to first ensure that you don't lose what you worked so hard to get. Here are some important keys to muscle maintenance:

- Keep weight training. Muscle growth isn't a do-it-and-forget-it proposition. Your muscles start shrinking after about 96 hours if they're not stressed—that's why your workouts have been spaced no more than 4 days apart. To maintain your gains, you must stay with a program at least as challenging as the Core Program.
- On the other hand, don't be afraid to take a week off. Yes, you'll lose some muscle, but it doesn't take nearly as long to get it back as it does to build it in the first place. In fact, taking a week off every 2 or 3 months is an important strategy. The break helps your muscles recover completely and rejuvenates your brain, too.
- When you come back from a break, return with a new routine. Your muscles stop adapting to the same

kind of stress after about 6 to 8 weeks of it. And even if you're content to maintain the level you're already at, more than 6 weeks of the same old stuff leads to less intensity, more boredom, and a consequent loss of strength and muscle mass.
- You don't have to increase sets or exercises beyond what you did in the Core Program. Ten exercises, 18 sets, and 45 minutes in the weight room three times a week is plenty. At times throughout the year you'll probably want to increase the volume and accelerate your gains. But to make steady progress toward a leaner, stronger, more muscular physique, the parameters set in the Core Program are fine.
- Intensity matters. You don't need to go all-out on every set you do for the rest of your life—in fact, that would be a bad idea—but you won't make gains if you don't challenge yourself continually with harder exercises, heavier weights, and more advanced techniques.

AEROBICS

In most cases, your best approach to aerobics during maintenance is to leave well enough alone. By now, you should be doing an hour and a half of aerobic work per week, spending 60 minutes of that time in your target heart-rate zone. Any less jeopardizes cardiovascular benefits. Much more makes it hard to continue building muscle mass.

If you're still looking to get bigger in the chest, upper back, and shoulders, get the most out of your aerobic days by incorporating sprint and interval training, if you haven't already. These easy-hard combinations that were presented in chapters 10 and 11 keep your aerobic work at the right level for a weight trainer—you'll attack your body's fat without jeopardizing its muscle.

Another excellent maintenance strategy is multi-mode training—that is, doing more than one kind of aerobic exercise per session.

Here's one way to do this: Start off with a 5-minute warmup on a treadmill, and then continue with 5 minutes in your target-heart-rate zone. Then, without resting, switch to a stationary bike for 10 minutes in your target zone. (You can even do intervals—1 minute hard, 1 minute easy for 10 minutes.) Finish with 10 minutes on the elliptical machine, the last 5 at a cooldown pace.

This offers at least three advantages: Your body is forced to continually adjust, rather than settle into a groove. The stress on your leg muscles is varied. And you discover why there's usually a line for the elliptical machine, if you haven't already.

EATING

The basic strategies from the Core Program will serve you well for maintenance. Keep your macronutrient ratio at 50 percent carbohydrates, 30 percent fat, and 20 percent protein. Avoid saturated fats in favor of mono- or polyunsaturated fats. And stay away from calorie-deficit weight-loss plans if you want to keep adding muscle mass.

The lifting and cardiovascular work you've been doing has probably cut down on your body fat. You may weigh the same (or more), but you're leaner.

If at some point you need to shed stubborn extra pounds more than you need to get even bigger in the chest and shoulders, cut down your calorie intake by no more than 500 calories a day, or 15 percent of your daily calorie intake, whichever is less. This will help ensure that the weight you lose is fat, not your hard-earned muscle mass. Keep your workouts at the same intensity, but don't expect to gain muscle size while you're losing weight. You may add a little lean mass, but it's a bonus if you do. Your first goal is to make sure you don't lose what you already have.

Whether you're still bulking up or trying to slim down, you want to eat five or six times a day, rather than the traditional three squares. For example, if you're trying to bulk up and you're eating 4,000 calories a day, you might have three 1,000-calorie meals and two 500-calorie snacks, with no more than 3 or 4 hours between meals. This will help you sustain a high energy level throughout the day, keep you from getting too hungry and gorging at any one meal, and allow you to exercise at any time of day without feeling bloated or malnourished.

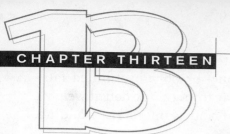

CHAPTER THIRTEEN

ESSENTIAL
ADVANCED
ROUTINES

Onward and upward. The 6-week Core Program has brought you to new levels of upper-body strength; now it's time for new challenges. This chapter offers five of them.

1. A hypertrophy (muscle-growing) program based on supersets.

2. An advanced routine focusing on strength rather than mass.

3. A sports routine designed to improve your performance as well as your upper torso.

4. A Swiss-ball workout, which improves your balance and coordination as well as increasing your muscle mass.

5. A one-exercise wonder for the shoulders.

HYPERTROPHY WORKOUT

Here's a challenging workout that delivers fast muscle growth via supersets—sets of two or more consecutive exercises with no rest in between. The exercises are presented in pairs based on the muscle group worked—two for the chest, two for the upper back, two for the shoulders.

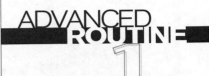

- Do a set of 8 to 12 repetitions of each exercise in the superset without pausing for any longer than it takes to move from one piece of equipment to the next.
- After each superset, rest 30 to 60 seconds. Then move on to the next. (You'll do each superset shown here once.)
- When you've finished a superset for each muscle group, rest 5 minutes. Then move on to the next three. Rest 5 minutes, then do the final three supersets.
- For the back exercises using one arm, do both exercises in the superset with one arm, then repeat the superset with the other arm.
- Do all nine supersets on Monday and Friday for 6 weeks.
- Change the order of the exercises every 2 weeks, but don't break up the pairs.

Decline Bench Press (Chest)

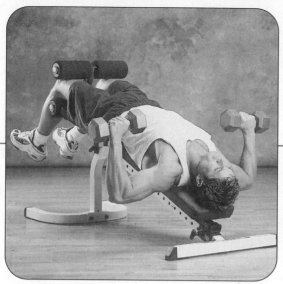
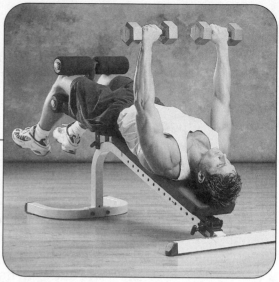

READY, SET:

Grab a pair of dumbbells and lie on your back on a decline bench with your head lower than your torso and your feet secured as shown. Hold the dumbbells on either side of your lower chest with your palms facing up and your elbows down. Make sure your back and head are firm against the bench.

GO:

Contracting your chest muscles, press the dumbbells upward and inward so they almost touch at the top of the movement. Pause, and slowly lower them back to the starting position.

PERFORMANCE TIPS

- The goal is to work the fibers of the lower chest harder than the fibers in the middle or upper chest. The steeper the angle of the decline bench, the more you'll emphasize these fibers.

- Make sure you maintain the same hand position throughout the movement and that your elbows come down outside your torso rather than scrunched against your sides. This emphasizes the pecs over the triceps.

- Keep your head and shoulder blades pressed against the bench throughout the movement, with a natural arch in your lower back. If you have to arch your lower back excessively to push the dumbbells up, you're using too much weight.

High-Cable Fly (Chest)

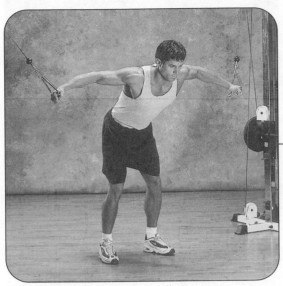 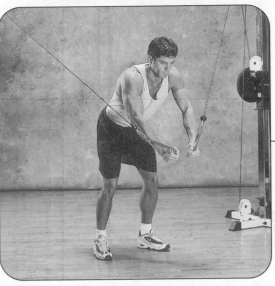

READY, SET:

Attach two stirrup handles to the high-cable pulleys in the cable-crossover machine and position yourself between the two weight stacks, bending forward at the waist 45 degrees. Hold the handles with your arms extended down and in front of you, your palms facing each other.

GO:

Slowly raise your arms out and up until they're parallel to the floor. Pause, and slowly pull the handles down to the starting position, tracing an upside-down semicircle in front of you.

PERFORMANCE TIPS

■ Your goal is to work the lower fibers of the pectoralis major. One way to ensure that you hit them is to pretend you're an old-time muscleman, showing off your spectacular chest to a crowd. Make sure your arms go below your chest, rather than crossing over in front of it—you wouldn't want to block it from your audience. The muscleman fantasy also helps you remember to keep your chest and arms tight throughout the movement.

■ Don't lock your elbows at any point—even at the fully extended position.

■ Pull your shoulders back at the start of the movement, and keep them back throughout the exercise. Although this shortens your range of motion, it helps protect your shoulders from injury and keeps the emphasis on your chest muscles rather than your shoulders.

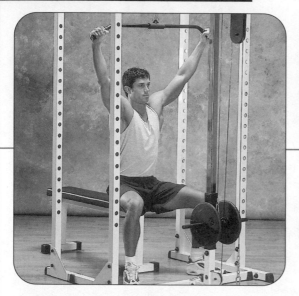
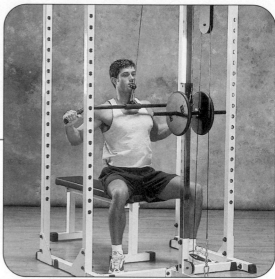

LAT PULLDOWN TO FRONT: Perform this exercise as you did in the Core Program. Using a wide overhand grip, bring the bar down to your chest.

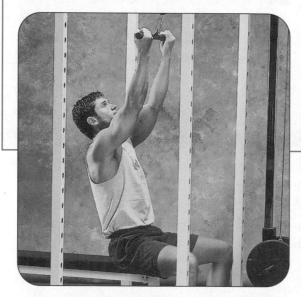
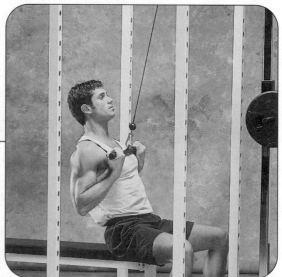

REVERSE-GRIP PULLDOWN: Perform this exercise as you did in the Core Program. Grab the bar with an underhand grip that's narrower than shoulder-width, and pull it down to the middle of your chest.

▲ *For more detailed instructions and performance tips for these exercises, see pages 65 and 81.*

Dumbbell Shoulder Press (Shoulders)

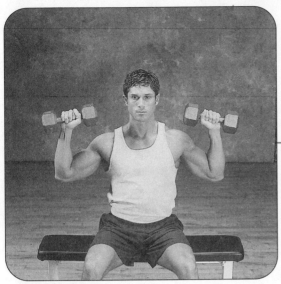 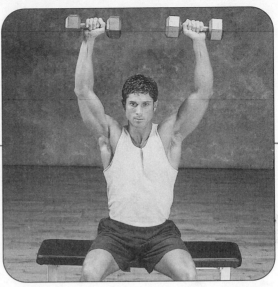

READY, SET:

Grab a pair of dumbbells and sit on the edge of a bench, holding the weights at shoulder level, your palms facing away from you. Push your chest out, pull your shoulders back, and focus your eyes straight ahead.

GO:

Push the dumbbells straight up over your head until your arms are straight. Pause, then lower the weights to the starting position.

PERFORMANCE TIPS

■ Keep your abdomen tight throughout the movement, and don't arch your back. In other words, maintain good posture.

■ Focus your mind on your deltoids, picturing them doing the lift, rather than your triceps.

■ Make sure your arms go up and not out. Don't rotate your shoulders or turn your grip as you go up or down.

■ You can perform this exercise standing. That makes it a little more challenging to your entire body, since there's more balance required, but also makes it easier to cheat and generate a little extra momentum with your lower body. Make sure you stand with your knees slightly bent and your back in its natural alignment, and keep your feet flat on the floor.

Front Raise (Shoulders)

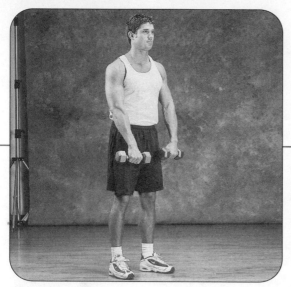 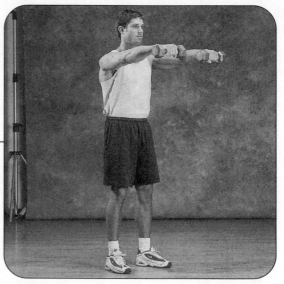

READY, SET:

Grab a pair of dumbbells and stand with your feet shoulder-width apart. Hold the dumbbells at arm's length in front of your legs, with your palms turned toward your front thighs. Bend your elbows slightly.

GO:

Lift the dumbbells straight up in front of you to about shoulder level. Pause, then slowly lower them to the starting position.

PERFORMANCE TIPS

■ It doesn't take a lot of weight to get a nice contraction in your front deltoids. Those are small muscles, and this is a finesse move, not a power exercise. A slow movement with light weights will help you more than a sloppy, jerky lift with heavier weights.

■ Lift the dumbbells in parallel arcs in front of you—don't let them stray out to the sides.

■ Your back plays a couple of important roles in this exercise. Your lower back is crucial for maintaining your postural stability as you raise objects out in front of you. And your shoulder blades rotate downward as you lift the weights, bringing various back muscles into the lift. These movements occur whether you think about them or not. The key is to keep your back upright and in its natural alignment throughout the exercise.

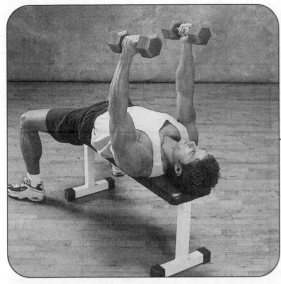 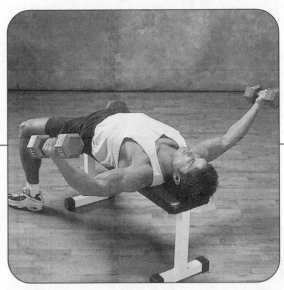

DUMBBELL FLY: Perform this exercise as you did in the Core Program. Hold a pair of dumbbells, your palms turned toward each other, as you lie on your back on a flat bench. Slowly lower the dumbbells until your upper arms are parallel to the floor, pause, then pull them back to the starting position.

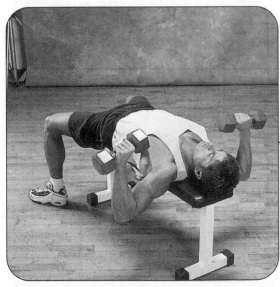 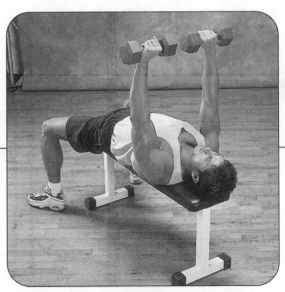

DUMBBELL BENCH PRESS: Perform this exercise as you did in the Core Program. Lie back on a flat bench and push two dumbbells up and toward each other from either side of your chest until your arms are extended.

▲ *For more detailed instructions and performance tips for these exercises, see pages 63 and 64.*

Barbell Bent-Over Row (Back)

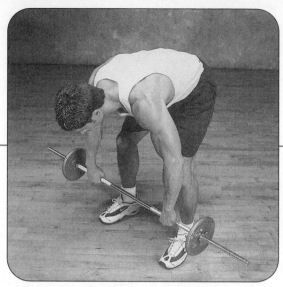
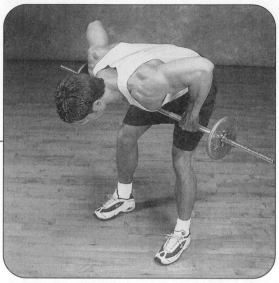

READY, SET:

Grab a barbell with an overhand, shoulder-width grip, and stand with your feet just less than shoulder-width apart. Bend your knees slightly, then bend forward at the hips between 45 and 90 degrees. The barbell should hang in front of you just below your knees. Pull your shoulder blades toward each other in back and tighten your entire torso.

GO:

Pull the barbell to your upper abdomen, pause, then slowly lower it back to the starting position.

PERFORMANCE TIPS

■ This exercise is one of the most popular mass-building upper-back exercises. In a hard-core gym, you'll see guys doing it with hundreds of pounds. You should approach it as a finesse exercise. Lift lighter weights slowly, trying to feel your upper-back and rear-shoulder muscles contracting.

■ Keep your legs and hips out of the lift. Your knees should stay slightly bent throughout, and your torso should maintain the same angle.

■ Your elbows should point to the ceiling at the top of the lift.

■ This is one of the riskiest exercises for your lower back, so you have to control the bar throughout the lift. Never jerk it up or let gravity take it down.

Seated Cable Row (Back)

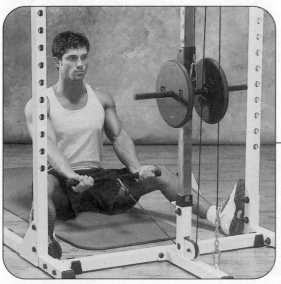
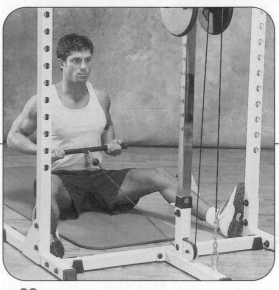

READY, SET:

Attach a straight bar to the low-cable pulley and position yourself in the apparatus with your feet against the platform. Grab the bar with an underhand grip, your hands just less than shoulder-width apart. Sit up straight with your shoulders back, arms and legs extended in front of you, and a slight bend in your elbows and knees.

GO:

Pull the bar to your abdomen, pause, then slowly return the bar to the starting position.

PERFORMANCE TIPS

- The key to this exercise is a full contraction in your middle- and upper-back muscles. Never return the bar to the starting position until you've felt a solid squeeze in those muscles.

- Your upper torso will want to lean back as you pull the bar in. But try to keep it from rocking back and forth during the movement.

- Relax your hands and arms. That will help you concentrate on pulling the bar with your upper-back muscles.

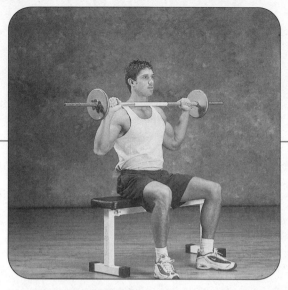 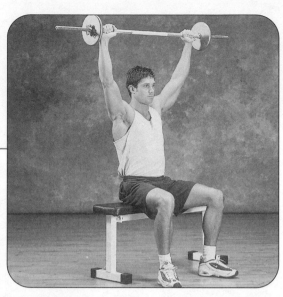

BARBELL SHOULDER PRESS: Perform the same movement as the dumbbell shoulder press (page 103), but use a barbell held with an overhand grip that's just wider than your shoulders.

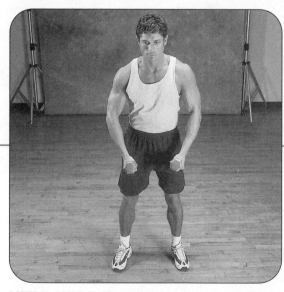 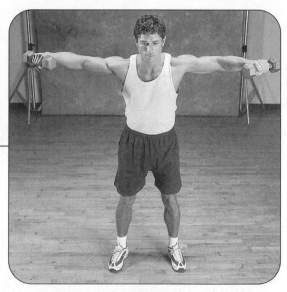

LATERAL RAISE: Perform this exercise as described on page 67. Raise two dumbbells out to your sides until your body makes a T.

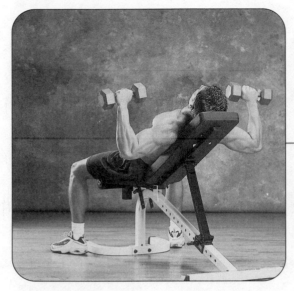 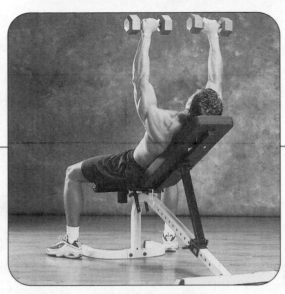

INCLINE DUMBBELL PRESS: Lie on your back on an incline bench and lift dumbbells straight up.

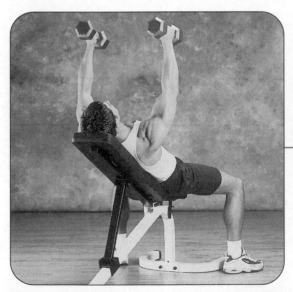 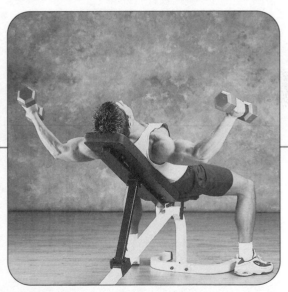

INCLINE DUMBBELL FLY: Grab a pair of dumbbells and lie on your back on an incline bench. Perform the exercise as you did on a flat bench in the Core Program.

▲ *For more detailed instructions and performance tips for these exercises, see pages 79 and 63.*

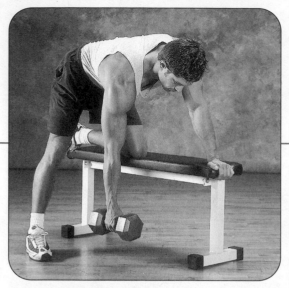 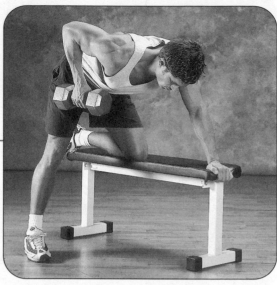

BENT-OVER DUMBBELL ROW: Perform this exercise as described on page 66 of the Core Program, but after finishing the repetitions with one arm, move directly to the next exercise in the superset (one-arm seated row). Do those repetitions with the same arm, then repeat the entire superset with the other arm.

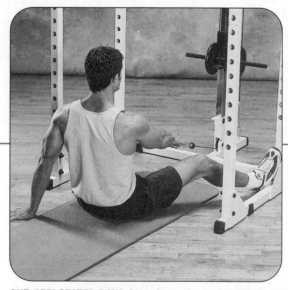 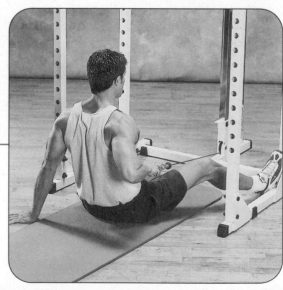

ONE-ARM SEATED ROW: Attach a stirrup handle to the low-cable pulley and position yourself in the rowing station. Grab the handle with an overhand grip, sit up straight, and pull your shoulders back. Start with your working arm extended, and your other arm braced against the floor behind you for balance. Pull the handle to the side of your abdomen, pause, then slowly return to the starting position.

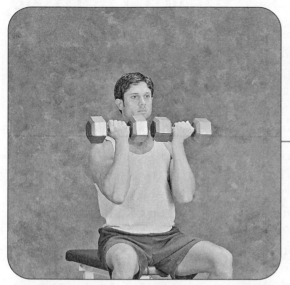
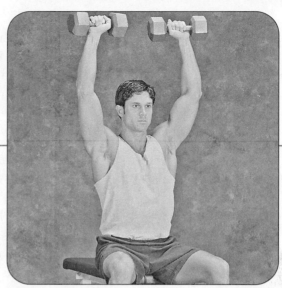

ROTATION PRESS: Perform this exercise as you did in the Core Program (page 53). Push a pair of dumbbells from under your chin straight up over your head, rotating your grip from palms in to palms out.

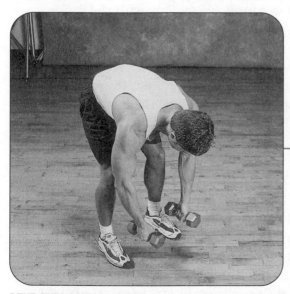
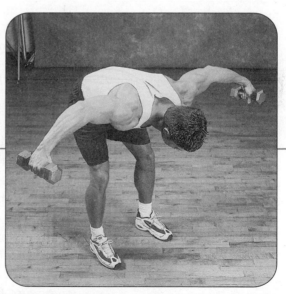

BENT-OVER LATERAL RAISE: Perform this exercise as you did in the Core Program. Bending forward at the hips, lift two dumbbells out the sides until your upper arms are parallel to the floor.

▲ *For more detailed instructions and performance tips for these exercises, see pages 68 and 83.*

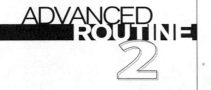

STRENGTH ROUTINE

Most of the exercises in this 6-week strength program will be familiar to you from the Core Program and the Hypertrophy Workout. However, the sets and rep counts are arranged to stress strength development more than muscle mass. Be forewarned: The volume's a tad higher than you're used to from the Core Program.

■ Do this routine on Monday and Friday.

■ For the first 2 weeks, do the first eight exercises—two for the chest, two for the back, four for the shoulders. Follow the set and rep counts provided.

■ During the 3rd and 4th weeks, switch to the next four chest and back exercises presented, following the set and rep counts given. Do the same four shoulder exercises (with more sets of the shoulder presses, using heavier weights for fewer reps).

■ During the 5th and 6th weeks, do the last four chest and upper-back exercises presented, following the set and rep counts given. Stay with the same four shoulder exercises (shifting sets and repetitions on the shoulder presses as described).

■ Where a time allotment (such as "60 seconds") replaces the repetition count for a set, the goal is to "flush" the muscle, clearing out the lactic acid accumulated during the previous sets. Choose a light weight and do repetitions for the time allotted.

■ Do one or two warmup sets of an exercise before multiple sets of eight or fewer reps. You don't have to warm up for the 60-second sets or an exercise in which you do more than eight reps.

■ Use the same weight on all sets of an exercise in a workout. Stop just short of "failure"—the point at which you can't do another rep with good form—on these sets. If the exercise calls for three sets of eight reps, use a weight you know you can do 10 times. By the final set, you should get near failure.

■ Rest 2 minutes between sets.

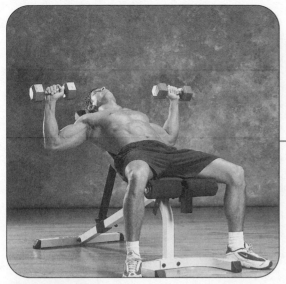 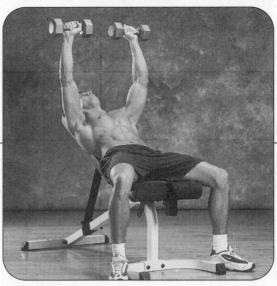

INCLINE DUMBBELL PRESS: Perform this exercise as described on page 79. Do three sets of eight reps in Weeks 1 and 2.

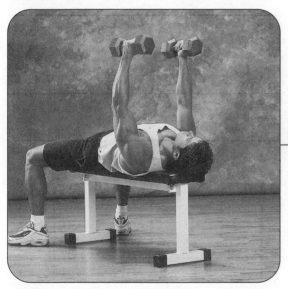 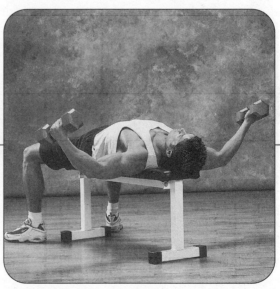

DUMBBELL FLY: Perform this exercise as described on page 63. Do two sets of 60 seconds each in Weeks 1 and 2.

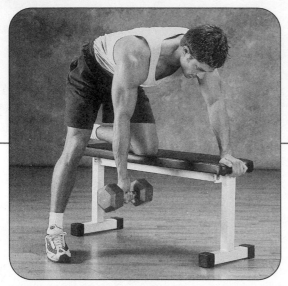 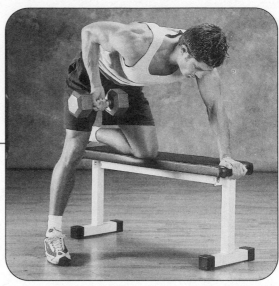

REVERSE-GRIP BENT-OVER ROW: Perform this exercise as described on page 66, changing to an underhand grip. Do three sets of eight reps in Weeks 1 and 2.

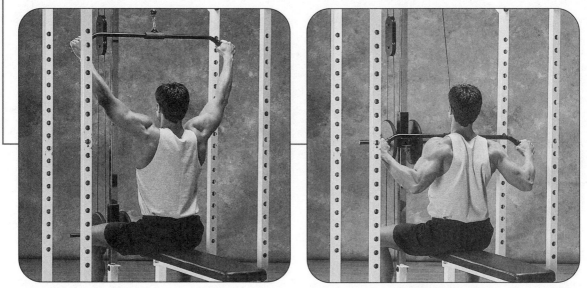

LAT PULLDOWN TO FRONT: Perform this exercise as described on page 65. Do three sets of eight reps in Weeks 1 and 2.

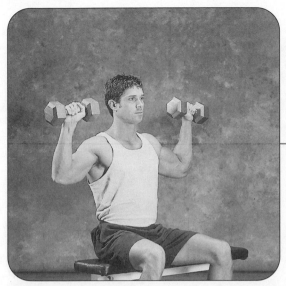 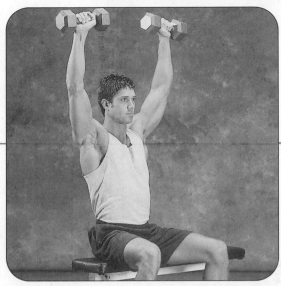

DUMBBELL SHOULDER PRESS: Perform this exercise as described on page 103. Or do the barbell version shown on page 108. Do three sets of eight reps in Weeks 1 and 2, four sets of five reps in Weeks 3 and 4, and five sets of three reps in Weeks 5 and 6.

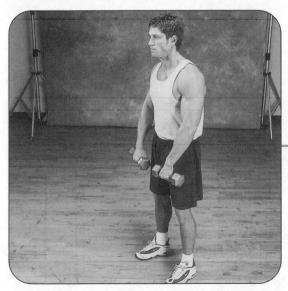 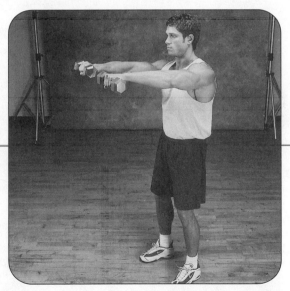

FRONT RAISE: Perform this exercise as described on page 104. Do one set of 15 reps throughout the program.

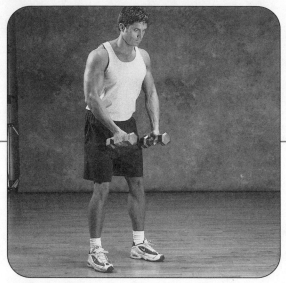
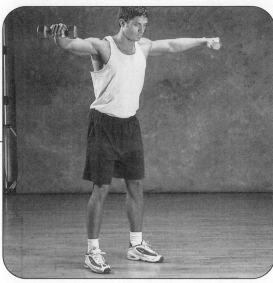

LATERAL RAISE: Perform this exercise as described on page 67. Do one set of 15 reps throughout the program.

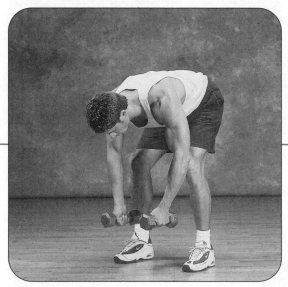
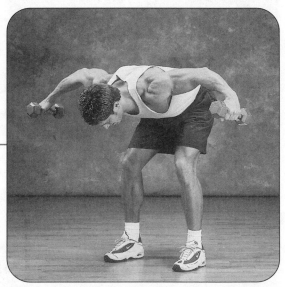

BENT-OVER LATERAL RAISE: Perform this exercise as described on page 83. Do one set of 15 reps throughout the program.

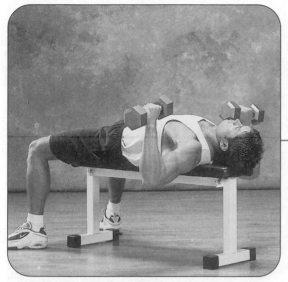
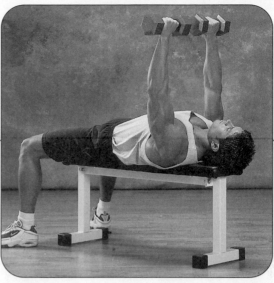

DUMBBELL BENCH PRESS: Perform this exercise as described on page 64. Do four sets of five reps in Weeks 3 and 4.

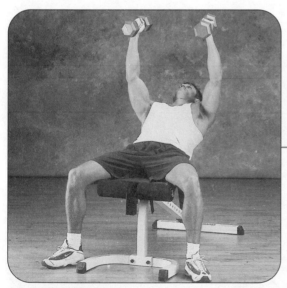
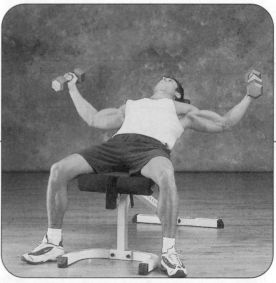

INCLINE DUMBBELL FLY: Perform this exercise as described on pages 63 and 109. Do two sets, the first at 60 seconds, the second at 90 seconds, in Weeks 3 and 4.

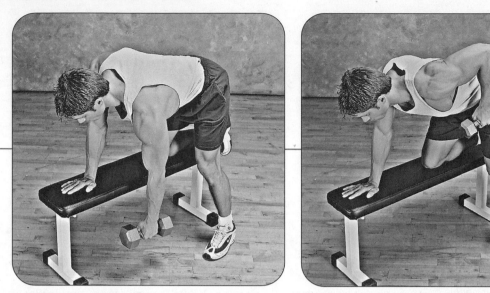

BENT-OVER DUMBBELL ROW: Perform this exercise as described on page 66. Do four sets of five reps in Weeks 3 and 4.

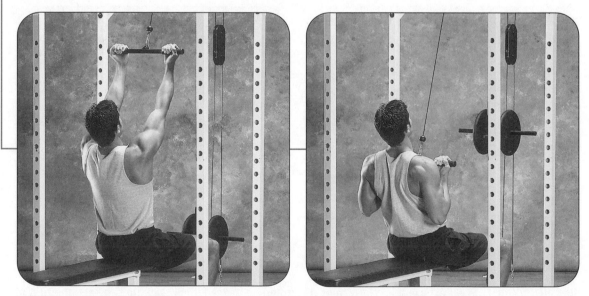

REVERSE-GRIP LAT PULLDOWN: Perform this exercise as described on page 81. Do three sets of eight reps in Weeks 3 and 4.

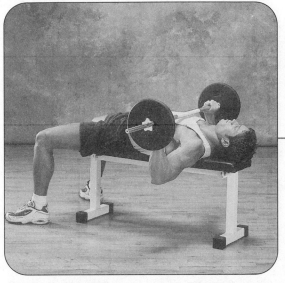
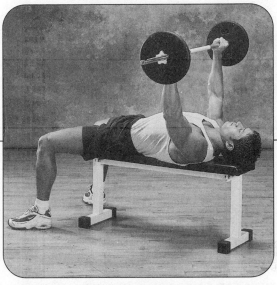

BARBELL BENCH PRESS: Lie on your back on a flat bench, grab the bar with an overhand grip that's just outside shoulder-width, and lift it from the uprights. Hold it over your chin at arm's length. Slowly lower the bar to your chest, pause, and push it back up. Do five sets of three reps in Weeks 5 and 6.

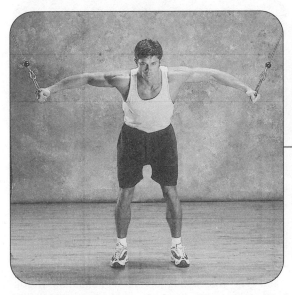
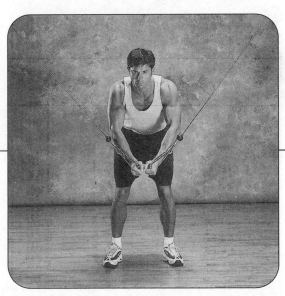

HIGH-CABLE FLY: Perform this exercise as described on page 101. Do two sets for 90 seconds each in Weeks 5 and 6.

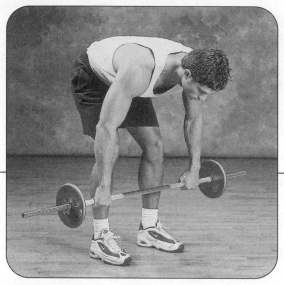 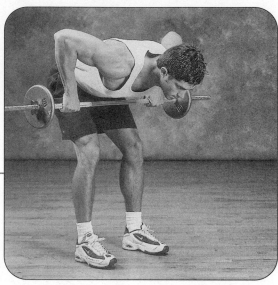

BARBELL BENT-OVER ROW: Perform this exercise as described on page 106. Do four sets of five reps in Weeks 5 and 6.

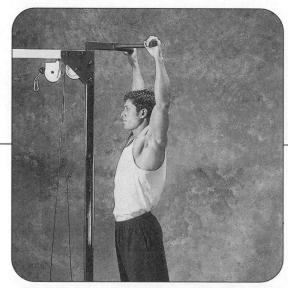 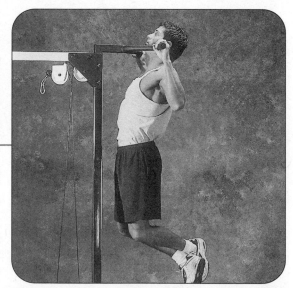

PULLUP: Jump up and grab the pullup bar with an overhand grip, your hands just outside shoulder-width. Hang from the bar with your knees bent and feet crossed behind you. Pull yourself up until your chin crosses the bar. Do three sets of eight reps, or to exhaustion.

SPORTS PERFORMANCE

Here's a 6-week program that will noticeably improve your game as well as your upper-body strength. The rotator-cuff muscles, key to so many sports, are emphasized.

- Do this workout on Monday and Friday.
- Rest 60 seconds between exercises the first 2 weeks, 90 seconds the next 2 weeks, and 2 minutes the last 2 weeks.
- During the first 2 weeks, do one set of 15 repetitions for each of the eight exercises.
- In Weeks 3 and 4, do two sets of 8 to 12 reps for all the exercises except the shoulder pushup. For that, do one set to exhaustion.
- In Weeks 5 and 6, do three sets of 6 to 10 reps for the chest and upper-back exercises. For the shoulders, do two sets of 6 to 10 reps of the internal and external rotation; three sets of 6 to 10 reps of the push press; and one set to exhaustion of the shoulder pushup.

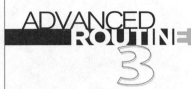

ADVANCED ROUTINE 3

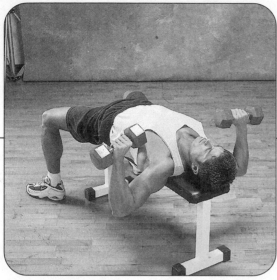
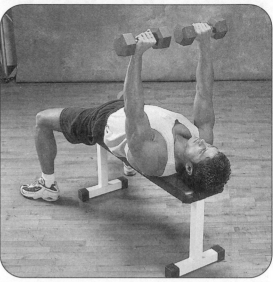

DUMBBELL BENCH PRESS: Do this exercise as described on page 64, but start from the extended (arms-up) position and do the movement with one arm at a time, alternating. So lower one dumbbell to the side of your chest, pause, push the dumbbell back up, then repeat with the other arm. That's one repetition.

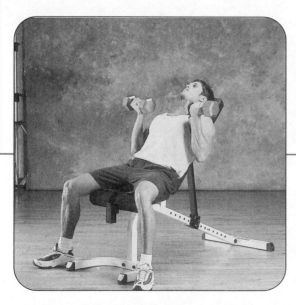
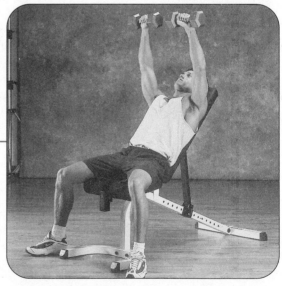

INCLINE ROTATION PRESS: Perform this exercise as described on page 68, but use an incline bench as shown, set at an angle of between 45 and 90 degrees.

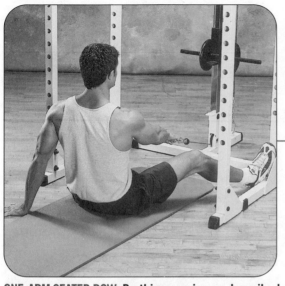 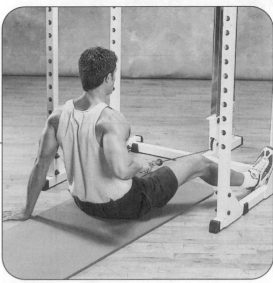

ONE-ARM SEATED ROW: Do this exercise as described on page 110.

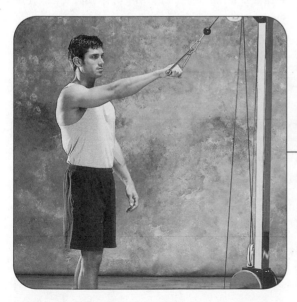 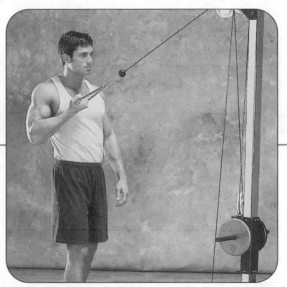

SINGLE-ARM ROTATION PULLDOWN: Attach a single handle to the high pulley, grab it with an overhand grip and pull it just below your chin, rotating the grip to underhand on the way down. Rotate the grip back again on the way up.

Internal Rotation (Shoulders)

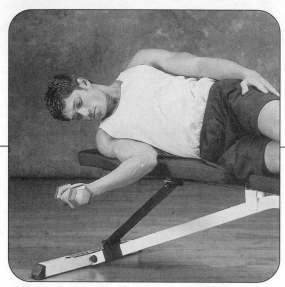 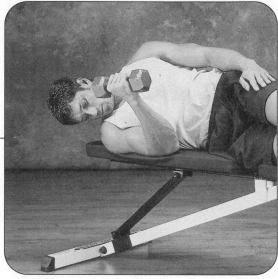

READY, SET:

Grab a dumbbell with your right hand and lie on your right side on a flat bench. Press your right upper arm and elbow against your side and along the edge of the bench, and bend the elbow 90 degrees so your right thumb points toward your head. Your right lower arm should be completely off the bench.

GO:

Rotate your shoulder to lower only your lower arm away from your body as far as comfortable. Pause, then lift weight up toward your chest as far as you can. Finish the set with your right arm, then repeat with your left.

PERFORMANCE TIPS

■ This shoulder movement emphasizes your rotator-cuff muscles, rather than the deltoids. You should feel the exercise on the inside front of your shoulder.

■ Use light weights and slow, careful movements. These are small, injury-prone muscles.

■ Keep your upper arm and elbow in a fixed position through the exercise.

External Rotation (Shoulders)

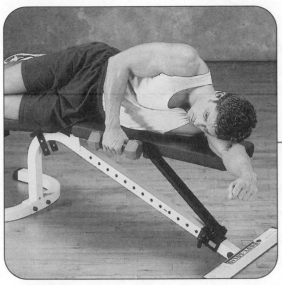 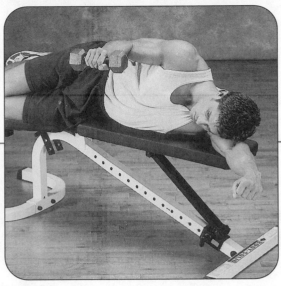

READY, SET:

Grab a dumbbell in your right hand and lie on your left side, resting your head on your extended left arm. Press your right upper arm and elbow against your right side. Your right elbow is bent 90 degrees, and your right lower arm lies across your torso.

GO:

Rotate your shoulder to raise the dumbbell toward the ceiling without moving your upper arm or elbow. Pause, then lower the weight to the starting position. Finish the set with your right arm, then repeat with your left.

PERFORMANCE TIPS

■ You should feel this exercise in the middle and back of your shoulder.

■ As with internal rotation, use light weights and slow movements. Your object with this exercise is to strengthen the muscles to prevent injury, not incur an injury by using too much weight or sloppy form.

Push Press (Shoulders)

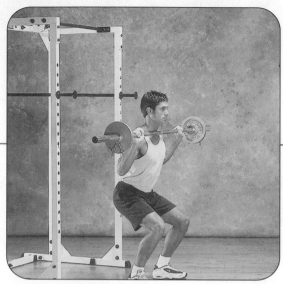 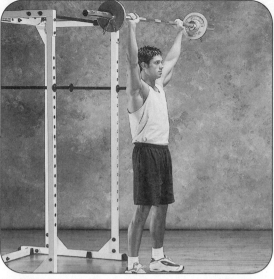

READY, SET:

Set a barbell on a squat or power rack at chest level. Grab the bar with an overhand grip that's wider than shoulder-width. Take the bar off the rack and rest it on your front shoulders; stand with your feet shoulder-width apart, your butt back and your knees bent in a quarter-squat position.

GO:

Bend your knees a bit more and immediately push the bar straight up over your head, using your legs, arms, and shoulders. Pause, then slowly return the bar to the starting position.

PERFORMANCE TIPS

■ This is an explosive movement, so do the lift faster than usual.

■ Though your delts and triceps do most of the work, you'll be pushing off with your legs at first. Think of jumping.

■ Keep your back in its natural alignment. Don't arch it excessively.

Shoulder Pushup (Shoulders and Triceps)

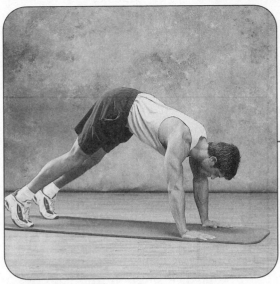 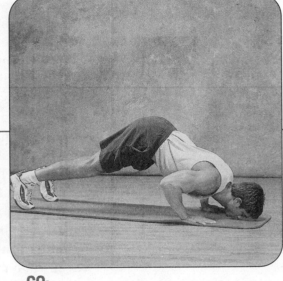

READY, SET:

Position yourself on your hands and toes so your body forms an arch. Your arms are fully extended and your hands and feet are just wider than shoulder-width apart.

GO:

Bend at the elbows and slowly lower your head to the floor. Pause, than push back up to the starting position.

PERFORMANCE TIPS

■ You can add a few inches to the range of motion if you lift your head at the end of the movement. But that could put extra strain on your shoulders. Try it both ways and see which version feels better.

■ If it's too easy on the floor, you can try it with your feet up on a bench, chair, or even a wall. The higher your feet are off the ground, the more resistance you'll get from gravity, and the harder the exercise will be.

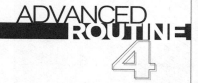

ADVANCED
ROUTINE
4

THE WELL-ROUNDED WORKOUT

Swiss balls. Resista-balls. Thera-balls. Stability balls. Call them what you will, these big, vinyl balls are increasingly common in gyms these days.

Their major advantage is to force your muscles to work in an unstable, 360-degree environment, rather than in the two-dimensional world of machines and benches. The balls are popular in the sports-training world and in injury rehabilitation because they build strength and muscle mass while teaching your muscles to work with each other, rather than in isolation.

For you, the benefits come from the new challenges to muscles that have developed nicely using the two-dimensional model. Now they'll have to move weights through a new range of motion while struggling to stay balanced. The greatest benefit may not come in actual size to your upper-torso muscles, but to your lower-torso muscles, which will have to work hard throughout the exercises to maintain balance.

Try this six-exercise Swiss-ball routine for 6 weeks. Do one set of 8 to 12 repetitions of each exercise the first 2 weeks. Do two sets in Weeks 3 and 4, and three sets in the final 2 weeks. Rest about 60 seconds between exercises.

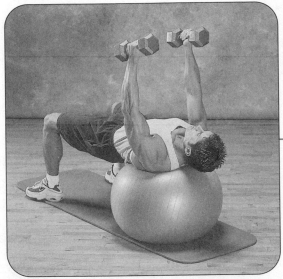
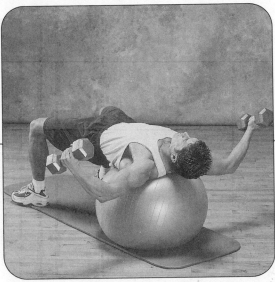

DUMBBELL FLY: Lying on the ball as shown, hold the dumbbells above your chest, your palms facing each other. Lower the weights until your upper arms are parallel to the floor. Pause, then lift the weights back to the starting position along the same arc.

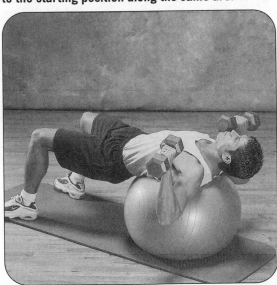
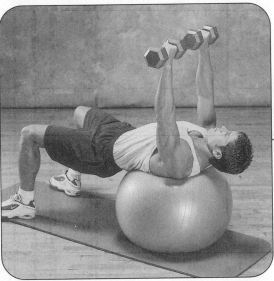

DUMBBELL PRESS: Grab a pair of dumbbells and lie on your back on the ball, with your feet flat on the floor and your head slightly higher than your chest. Hold the dumbbells outside your shoulders with your palms facing the ceiling. Push the weights up and toward each other until your arms are fully extended. Pause, then slowly lower them to the starting position.

▲ *More detailed instructions and performance tips for the standard versions of these exercises are on pages 63 and 64.*

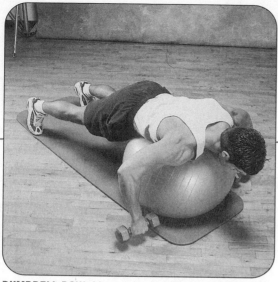 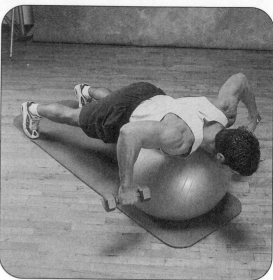

DUMBBELL ROW: Lie on your chest on a ball, your toes on the floor. Hold the dumbbells with your elbows out and palms facing behind you. The dumbbells should be as close to the floor as you can get them without them actually resting on it. Pull your shoulder blades together in back and lift your head so your neck is in alignment with your back. Now pull the weights up until your upper arms are parallel to the floor.

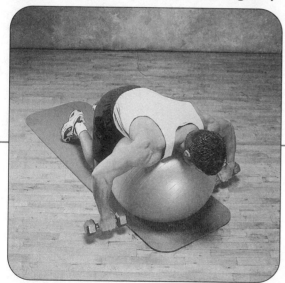 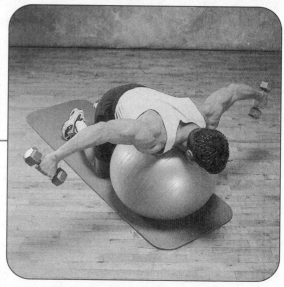

BENT-OVER LATERAL RAISE: Kneel with your chest on the ball. Hold the dumbbells straight down from your shoulders, with your palms facing backward and elbows bent slightly. Lift the dumbbells straight out to the sides, pause, then slowly return to the starting position.

▲ *More detailed instructions and performance tips for the standard versions of these exercises are on pages 52 and 83.*

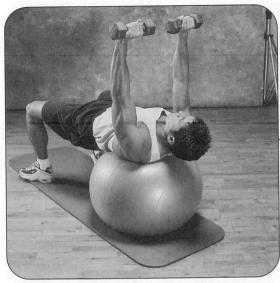 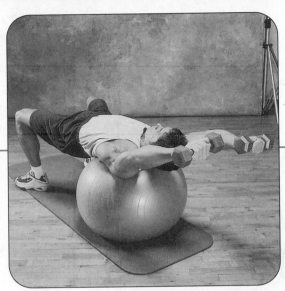

DUMBBELL PULLOVER: Grab a pair of dumbbells and lie on your back on the ball, your feet on the floor and your head at the same level as your chest. Hold the dumbbells above your head with your palms facing the ceiling and elbows slightly bent. Slowly lower the weights behind your head until your upper arms are parallel to the floor.

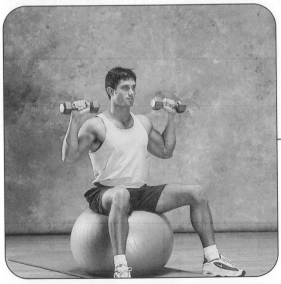 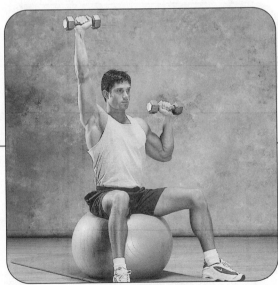

ALTERNATING DUMBBELL SHOULDER PRESS: Hold the dumbbells at the sides of your shoulders, palms facing out. Push one dumbbell straight up, pause, then slowly lower it to the starting position and repeat with the other arm.

▲ *More detailed instructions and performance tips for the standard version of this exercise are on page 103.*

AROUND THE WORLD

When you don't have time to do a full shoulder workout, this one-exercise wonder comes in handy. With a single exercise, you can put your shoulder joint through a variety of motion, stimulating all three parts of the deltoid muscle.

Use a weight that will allow you to do 10 repetitions. Do all the movements in a slow, smooth and controlled manner.

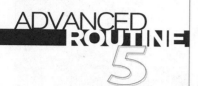

ADVANCED ROUTINE 5

AROUND THE WORLD

Around the World (Shoulders)

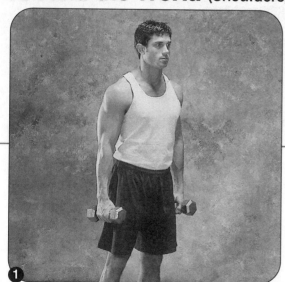

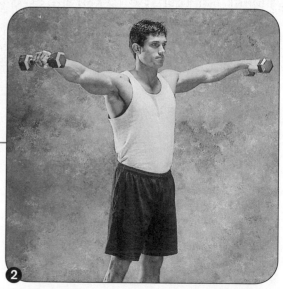

① READY, SET:
Hold two dumbbells at your sides with your palms facing each other and your elbows slightly bent.

② GO:
Raise the dumbbells to your sides, performing a lateral raise.

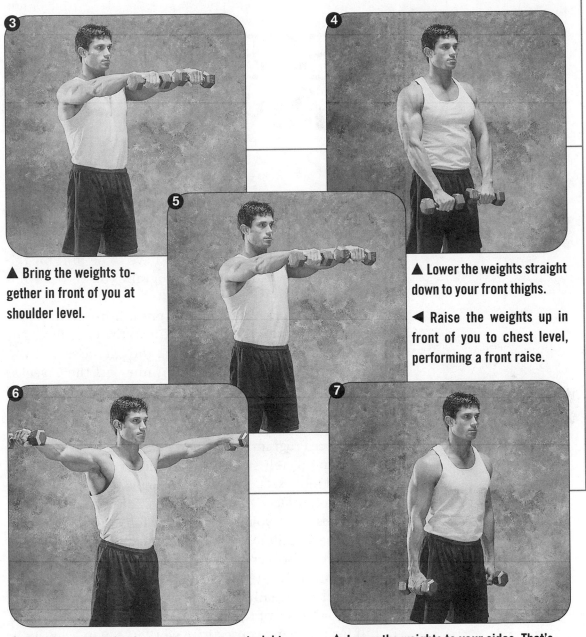

▲ Bring the weights to-
gether in front of you at
shoulder level.

▲ Lower the weights straight
down to your front thighs.

◀ Raise the weights up in
front of you to chest level,
performing a front raise.

▲ Pull the weights back, so your arms are straight
out to your sides again.

▲ Lower the weights to your sides. That's
one repetition.

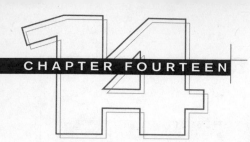

CHAPTER FOURTEEN

ESSENTIAL LONG-RANGE PLAN

By now you realize that achieving and then maintaining a great physique—particularly one that comes equipped with a V-shaped torso—is a lifelong project. So if you're in it at all, you have to be in it for the long run. Too bad the Core Program you've been following isn't.

Genetics and common sense put a limit on any progressive program. Let's say you finish the Core Program and don't want to quit—you like the exercises and the workout parameters. So you continue past the 6 weeks, adding more sets. Maybe that works for another couple of weeks—you see some gains in strength and muscle mass, but they aren't as dramatic as what you saw during the 6-week Core Program. So you add more. That doesn't help—you're completely stuck. In a final act of desperation, you add still more sets. Your workouts now take an hour and a half to complete. And for all that effort, you find you're lifting less than you did in the previous weeks, and your physique doesn't look as good, either.

You've discovered some of the basic rules of weightlifting. First, more isn't always better. Sometimes it is, but eventually you see diminishing returns. That leads to the law of plateaus: If you try to climb the same hill for too many consecutive workouts, you eventually discover there's no more hill to climb. If you're lucky, you end up on a plateau. You aren't making improvements anymore, but you aren't doing any worse. But most of us, at one time or another, find ourselves so hell-bent to keep going in a favorite workout program that we hit the top of the hill and never realize it until we find we're going downhill—losing strength, coming into the weight room with less energy than before, and either losing muscle or gaining fat, if not both.

These peaks, plateaus, and backslides seem inconceivable when you start a great new program. Each time, you think you're going to beat all the laws of human physiology and keep making gains forever. If this were possible, used-car lots would be full of 400-pound men deadlifting SUVs.

A beginner can get away with following the same program for 6 to 8 weeks. An intermediate lifter may not see gains after doing the same workout six times. Some advanced lifters have to change their workouts every time they go into the gym if they want to see any improvements at all. These guys never do the exact same workout twice.

The physiological reasons for all this are contained in the general adaptation syndrome, which was first formulated in the 1930s. Here's a capsule summary.

The alarm stage. Remember that soreness you felt after your first Core Program workout? That's your body's way of saying, "Whoa, something radical's going on here." Your training goal at the alarm stage is to get through it, to survive. I designed the Core Program with the idea that the initial shock to your body shouldn't be so great that you say "To hell with this" and toss *Essential Chest & Shoulders* into the "free" box outside the library.

The resistance stage. Instead of bagging the program, you made it to the next stage, and you reaped the benefits. In the resistance stage, your muscles adapt to the overload of resistance training by getting bigger and stronger. Your mechanics—your form on the exercises—improve as your muscles and nervous system work together with increasing efficiency. The self-confidence you gain from seeing results inspires you to train more intensely for even better gains in strength and muscle mass.

The exhaustion stage. All good things must end. This lesson applies to weight lifters as well as stock-market types who saw dot-com investing as an instant retirement plan. In the exhaustion stage—also called the overwork stage—your muscles stop responding to the same old sources of stress. Now you've hit a plateau, or perhaps even a regression.

You probably won't recognize this stage right away. You think you should still be making gains, and get frustrated when you don't. Your confidence slips. Your motivation isn't what it used to be. You start to notice some nagging little injuries, and some days you're tired before you even walk into the gym.

If you keep going after you hit this part of the training cycle, you'll push your body into what's called overtraining, which has a laundry list of nasty consequences: poor sleep, lethargy, weak appetite, chronic infections or illnesses.

Then there's the cruelest punishment of all: lost strength and muscle mass.

Life would be wonderful if we could be in the resistance stage each time we walked into the gym, and never hit the exhaustion stage. Though that's not physiologically possible, you can spend more time in the resistance stage than you currently do if you make frequent changes in your training program. This means more frequent wake-up calls from the alarm stage, but those sore, confused muscles are the harbinger of the strong, coordinated body you'll continue to develop.

CHANGE-UP STRATEGIES

You aren't going to change your workout completely every month or two. No one trains like that. You just need to make more subtle changes on a regular basis. Here are a few classic techniques.

Find a new slant. Do bench exercises at different grades of incline or decline. The higher you set the bench for dumbbell presses, for instance, the more you emphasize the upper pectorals and front shoulders over the middle and lower parts of your chest.

Vary the grip. A simple pullup—the best of all upper-back exercises—can become three different exercises if you shift from a wide overhand grip to a more narrow underhand grip to a neutral grip in which your palms are facing each other and just a few inches apart. The wider grip puts the most stress on your upper-back muscles. When you switch from overhand to underhand, you put your arms in a stronger position, so your biceps do more of the work and your back muscles a little less. Finally, the narrow grip means your chest picks up some work, and your arms are in their strongest position when they face each other.

Shift the angle. You've already discovered this technique in the Core Program. A simple lateral raise for your shoulders becomes three different exercises when you lift to the front, sides, or back.

Change speeds. Speeding up or slowing down the exercises makes a difference. We've already told you the effect of keeping your muscles under tension for 4 to 6 seconds per repetition, instead of the 2 or 3 seconds most guys use. Your muscles will get more sore at first, but they'll also get bigger faster. Sometimes, though, it pays to shift to faster repetitions using more weight. Your muscles are designed to work at different speeds, and if you always train them at the same speed with the same type of load, you won't hit all the muscle fibers that have the potential to grow bigger.

On the other hand, some trainers advocate going even slower, using reps of 10 to 20 seconds. This might prompt some immediate gains, since any new challenge to your muscles will result in quick growth. But it's not a long-term strategy. Your body will eventually get used to it, and you end up using the same muscle fibers over and over again to lift the weights slowly. Your high-threshold muscle fibers—the ones with the greatest potential for growth—won't get used at all. Plus, lifting slowly teaches your muscles to move slowly.

Go negative. The greatest muscle damage occurs when you lower a weight, resisting gravity. Since this is a well-accepted physiological principle, some guys figure that if a little emphasis on the negative portion of the repetition is good, a major emphasis must be better. So instead of a standard set using between 60 and 90 percent of the weight you could lift once with good form, you start with a weight that's heavier than your maximum lift—perhaps as much as 120 percent of it—and do a series of three or four negative reps, getting assistance on the lift and then lowering the weight as slowly as you can. (You can also use this technique at the end of a regular set, when your muscles are fried and can't do any more reps with good form.)

Obviously, this technique requires more caveats and qualifications than just about any you'll ever try. (I'm half-tempted to withhold the rest of the information until you sign a form releasing me from all liability.) First, you have to know going in that your muscles are probably going to get very sore. You also have to understand that it's a very quick leap from the alarm to the exhaustion stages, with hardly any time spent in resistance. That's how powerful this technique is. Three weeks is probably the absolute upper limit for training with negative reps. One or two workouts might be more realistic.

Safety is paramount. You have to be an experienced lifter with well-trained muscles—that means at least a year or two of consistent strength training, with serious gains to show for it. Then you either have to have an equally experienced training partner to help you, or use equipment that allows you an escape route. For negative bench presses, someone has to help you lift the weight. But you can also do them on a chest-press machine with a foot pedal that allows you to use your lower body to get the weight moving. Pullups are a good exercise for negative reps, since you can let go of the bar at the end of a repetition and climb back up to start the next one. Any exercise that puts stress on your lower back—such as a barbell bent-over row—is a bad idea. Try it and you'll quickly realize the multiple meanings of the word "negative."

Other rep restylings. A further rep-warping technique is extended pauses. Finish a rep and take several seconds to rest before the next one.

Finally, there's the "static contraction" method, which is a great one to use if you're pressed for time and can only do one set of each exercise. When you get to the final repetition in a set—you absolutely can't do one more with good form—you hold your muscles in the fully contracted position for as long as you can. This is a terrific technique to use on arm exercises. Again, you don't want to try this on an exercise that puts your back in a vulnerable position, such as the barbell bent-over row mentioned above.

WORKOUT OPTIONS

Besides varying the movements, there are lots of ways to arrange your sessions in the gym to confuse your muscles so that they keep making adaptations resulting in more strength and mass.

Reorder things. Working large muscles first and small muscles last is the generally preferred sequence, but it's not written in stone. Try mixing up the order you do the exercises from time to time. Sets of bench presses at the end of a workout instead of the beginning will hit your pecs at a far different state of fatigue. And working smaller muscles like your arms and shoulders first can result in bigger gains, since they won't be taxed from assisting with chest and back exercises.

Vary your rest periods. The Core Program recommends 30 to 60 seconds of rest between sets. To vary the mix, you might try taking longer breaks—90 to 120 seconds, for example. That allows you to approach each set with more intensity, lift more weight for more repetitions, and see bigger gains. Powerlifters might take 5 minutes between their heaviest sets. The only downside to the longer rest periods is that you limit the fat-burning properties of the workout. But you make up for it with bigger, stronger muscles.

Switch equipment. You can do most exercises with dumbbells, a barbell, cables, or any of several machines found in good gyms. You can create even more variations by switching from high to low cables, or from a straight bar to an EZ-curl bar (that's the shorter, cambered bar). Serious gyms also have bars that come in different thicknesses. A thicker bar is harder to grip, so you increase your hand and forearm strength when you use one. Finally, you can also do most of the popular exercises on a Swiss ball. That introduces a balance component, and brings midsection muscles in on upper-body exercises.

Do supersets. You may recall these consecutive sets of different exercises with no rest between them from the hypertrophy workout (page 99). Usually, a superset is two exercises for opposite muscle groups—a bench press followed by a seated row, for example. Two straight sets of exercises working the same muscle (fly, dumbbell bench press) is sometimes called a compound set. Three exercises in a row is a triset, and more than three in a row is called a giant set. The goal is the same with each—to work the muscles with increasing levels of exhaustion. The traditional superset, which works opposite muscles, also saves time, since one muscle can recover while the other is working.

NEW PROGRAMS

At some point, you're going to have to switch to an entirely new program to stay out of the exhaustion stage. Again, there are many good options:

High-volume versus high-intensity. The Core Program emphasizes intensity over volume, meaning you work harder on a limited number of sets rather than pacing yourself through a longer workout. That's the ideal approach in typical situations, especially if you're a beginner, returning from an injury, or concentrating on maintenance. But higher-volume workouts (20 to 30 total sets, say) have their place. Extremely advanced lifters might do 10 sets of 10 repetitions of an exercise to shock their muscles into new growth. Conversely, a guy who typically does 3 or 4 sets of every exercise will probably make terrific gains if he switches to one all-out set of each exercise.

The two schools aren't mutually exclusive. Most experienced lifters use a combination of high-volume and high-intensity techniques within each workout. So a guy might do four sets of bench presses, but just one set of an abdominal exercise.

Strength versus mass. "Strength training" is often used synonymously with "muscle building," as in this book. But the two are different (though obviously overlapping) pursuits. Whether a weight program emphasizes strength, muscle mass, or muscular endurance is largely determined by the repetitions. Low-rep sets (3 to 5, for example) are associated with strength development, with only modest increases in muscle size. Moderate repetitions (6 to 12) are ideal for bulking up, with some gains in strength. And higher reps (13 to 20) yield muscular endurance with little improvement in either strength or size. And even within these parameters, there's a lot of variance from one guy to the next. A guy who's been lifting for years might not see size increases unless he does low reps, whereas a beginner will probably see his strength and size improve with higher repetitions.

New directions. The advanced routines presented in chapter 13 offer some completely new programs for long-range development of your chest, arms, and shoulders. The day may come, though, when you want to emphasize another area of your body while maintaining your upper-torso gains. Two previous books in this series—*Essential Abs* and *Essential Arms*—provide programs to do just that.

GIVE YOURSELF A BREAK

The last essential element of your long-range training plan is to take periodic breaks from lifting. Just because training success is based on progressive effort, it doesn't mean a relentless march forward. Advances come in cycles. A week off after 6 weeks of hard training, or at the completion of a program, is vital for muscle recovery and prevention of both injury and burnout.

Regular breaks also help you keep your perspective. Your hours in the gym are important, but so are your family, friends, work, and play.

Remember, you're following a training program so it can improve your life—not take it over.

INDEX

Underscored page references indicate boxed text.
Boldface references indicate photographs.